LEARN *to* LISTEN
Your body is trying to talk to you

by Kevin McDonald

First published in New Zealand in 2009 by Kevin McDonald.
Printed by Zenith Print, New Plymouth, New Zealand,
assisted by PublishMe.co.nz

Design by Matt McDonald.

ISBN 978-0-473-15045-7

Dedication

This book is dedicated to my Dad and Mum.
Dad taught us all how to work
And the true value of hard work.

Mum, your gift of patience is something I will treasure
And be eternally thankful for.
Thanks for the gift of life
And all the gifts of the Spirit you have shown us.

CONTENTS

INTRODUCTION

It is with excitement as well as frustration that I start writing this book. I am really excited to finally find the time and head space to put down in words my thoughts on human health. The frustration is something I have had for many years. It is very frustrating to continually see so many unhealthy people coming to me for help because they have not been successful in their endeavours to find out what is wrong. Nor do they know why they have their particular condition. They are living each day in pain, discomfort, tiredness or general unwellness, yet I know for most of them they don't have to be that way. Many have been clearly diagnosed with a specific health condition, given a name for this condition, but still do not know why they have got it, nor what to do to get rid of their problem. So many are daily taking medications and supplements but not improving. Large numbers are taking supplements, exercising and working very hard on their dietary options but all to no avail. My frustration is because I know that most of the time there are very simple solutions to their problems.

The book title 'Learn to Listen' is something we all need to do. It has been said that intuition is our inner teacher. The human body does know how to talk to us but not in a language that we can always understand. When we break an ankle the body will talk very clearly. It will give severe pain in the ankle area so that we will know something is seriously wrong. There are many times though when the body will be sending us very strong messages but we don't know how to interpret them. Just what do those signals mean? We haven't learnt the full vocabulary of the body. Or is it that the body has not learnt to talk in our language, in a language that we can clearly and quickly understand. Oh, how many times have we had strong messages from the body for many years and not understood what they were? Both individually and collectively we need to learn how to listen more closely. The body does tell us when something is not right, and it will not lie to you when something is wrong with your health.

The excitement for me is that for many years I have seen simple things change the health of many people in ways that they thought were beyond them. It is rewarding for me when my clients are feeling the best they have for many years and comment that they actually have a life back now, yet have only had to do simple things to achieve this improvement.

What I hope to achieve with this book is to inform you the reader of what I believe is important with the functions of the human body. If you can read this book with an open mind I am sure you will see that the commonsense (or should I say logical-sense) approach I have in relation to our body functions will be relevant in your life. There is a lot of information about health available to us around the world mainly in books and on the internet. A lot of this information is correct and true, and most of it is very interesting, with great technical detail. However, the big challenge for us all is to find out which information is relevant to us. Some of the information we can get about any health issues are very interesting and intriguing to the point that we can get completely absorbed by it. All our efforts are sometimes put into a particular theory or practise that may be true but is just not relevant to our situation.

It is very hard for most of us to work out what is relevant for us rather than just what sounds right. Rule number one is, if you have a health problem do something about it. It's that simple. If you have got a problem do something. Most of the time if you do nothing, there will be no improvements. Rule number two is, if you give something a good try and you don't feel a significant change in your symptoms within 30 days, try something else. Don't repeat the same thing over and over if you are not getting the desired result. I know that when you are doing the right thing you will get a very clear change, well within 30 days. Most of the time there will be more than one solution to any given problem so don't let anyone tell you they have the only solution. Some practitioners will tell you that you will need to stick with the solution for 6 months or more before you will get an improvement. This may be correct, but I am sure there will be other things you could do that will give a good result in a shorter time frame.

So be proactive and hunt for the things you need to do to get your health up to a level that feels good for you. I trust that there will be things of interest in this book that you can resonate with. There may also be some things that are a bit challenging to your beliefs. Just because something is interesting does not mean it is true. In the same way, just because something is different to your long held beliefs does not mean it is false. What I ask is for you to read this book with an open mind and see if it sounds like logical commonsense. I make no apologies for the simple way in which I have explained some of the health issues I see. Look for simplicity. The answer will be there.

The information I share is just a small collection of the information I have picked up over the last 20 years of dealing with everyday normal human beings who are themselves looking for solutions to everyday health problems. I have received this information from thousands of different people and now share it with you and trust that you will further share it with others. I was taught how to listen and then I learnt how to listen at a deeper level. This book is a reflection of what I have heard from many human bodies over many years.

Take a risk. Learn to listen and happy reading.

Kevin.

Times and circumstances change. What may have been a reasonable solution yesterday, a valid position last month may not be tenable at all today. Indeed, life is a moving train and what was only a second ago will never be again.

Everyday we should all arise and ask ourselves three questions;

1. *Do I really want to know the truth about everything, or do I just want to confirm that the notions I already have about life are correct?*
2. *When I confront a new fact, am I willing to lay aside the convictions of a lifetime long enough to give this new information an opportunity to change my point of view?*
3. *Have I ever surrendered my most cherished opinions completely to an objective examination in hopes of finding out why I hold such views in the first place? Can I surrender my mind to the acceptance of the truth, regardless of whether that acceptance might create a hell on earth for me or lead me to heaven?*

One should never obsessively look back to see what he or she might have said about something in the past, but rather should keep his or her mind tuned to the truth of the present.

James M. Carroll, Knoxville, Tennessee.

THE HUMAN BODY

The body is a mirror of heaven;
Its energy makes angels jealous.
Rumi

The human body is a very complicated thing. Science has been able to work out many of the functions of the body and is continually discovering new aspects about it, but from my understanding there are a small number of very important things that are not yet clearly understood by science. Because of this it has become a case of "we can't see the forest because of the trees". In some areas of health we are completely missing the obvious. We don't know what we don't know so therefore we won't know that we don't know it.

I will endeavour to keep this information as simple as possible, in a form that will make a lot of common sense, and logical. I will not confuse you with complicated scientific terminology. There are many issues with human health that we have over complicated. We are looking for complex solutions when we should be going back to basics and looking for simple solutions. There is a principle called Occam's razor that states; "the best solution to a problem is almost always the simplest solution." I have seen this principle at work over many years with most of the people I deal with. In most cases the solutions are very simple and easy and usually give very clear significant improvements to a person's health situation.

In my work there are three main issues I see on a very regular basis that are the core underlying reasons why humans are unwell or not able to reach their full potential. These are:
1. Very poor digestion
2. Poor kidney function
3. Poor liver function

The end result of having one or more of these problems is the fact that there will not be enough quality nutrients getting to your cells so as to allow those cells to do their full function.

There are many other serious issues that people are dealing with on a daily basis but most of them will stem from the fact that either their digestion has been poor for many years, they have had long term liver problems, partly because the liver is our emotional centre and we have all had to deal with big emotional issues from time to time, or the fact that their kidney function is poor. The main function of the kidneys is to filter rubbish out of the body. If the efficiency of the kidneys is poor the consequences are very bad. The biggest concern with kidneys is that to my knowledge there is not one test anywhere on this planet that can tell you whether your kidneys can filter your rubbish out of your body. Numerically this is a very big problem, with serious side effects that are a major contributing factor in most of our common degenerative diseases.

I will cover these three main issues in some detail in the following chapters. What it all comes down to is whether your cells can get all the nutrients they require so as to be able to do their function well and then collectively these cells work together to make the whole body function fully. All cells need feeding; they need oxygen; they need their rubbish and toxins removed; they need quality sleep time so as to repair and replicate; and they need exercise and happiness. When they get these basic requirements in full measure they can function fully. It really is that simple.

We commonly hear that many of our diseases are because of our genetic make-up; it was passed on from our parents. For me this is only partly true and a very small contributing factor with health issues. Our genetic make-up may be similar to our parents and they may have a genetic disposition to get a particular disease or condition, which is then passed to the next generation, but from my experience it will nearly always take something within your cellular environment to trigger that genetic susceptibility. We will not get the health problem just because we have the same weak gene our parents had.

Chemicals have been shown to play a big part in many degenerative diseases that are prevalent in society today. Chemicals can do a large amount of damage at the cellular level and right down at the DNA level. However, in most cases it is very hard for a chemical to get into a cell and do any damage if that cell is fully fed with all the appropriate nutrients and antioxidants. A healthy well fed cell is a very strong resilient cell. The environment inside our cell will have a greater effect on our health than the effect our genetic make-up will have.

The human body, when looked at as a physical object, is nothing more than a collection of vitamins, minerals and nutrients that all work together in perfect harmony to allow life to happen. It is an amazing object that has many different energies and energy flows, yet all it needs is a steady supply of more of those nutrients from living plants to keep it functioning for many decades. If things are going well it has the ability to self replicate, repair and reproduce. It does it for us. We just need to do the right things and then let life happen rather than try to hard to make life happen. Our body is a wonderful thing to live in.

Now let's take a look at some of the common problems I see everyday that are seriously interfering with the ability of the body to be at its optimum level of function.

CHAPTER TWO
FOOD

What we eat and drink today,
Will make us walk and talk tomorrow.
Anonymous.

Simply put the main point of eating food is to keep the human body alive. While we do need oxygen to keep alive, because if we don't get enough oxygen we hit the floor pretty fast, the next most important thing after oxygen is food and water. I would regard water as a food as it nourishes our cells. A lot of nutrients can and should arrive into our body through water.

There are approximately one hundred trillion cells in a human body made up of about 200 different cell types. Every cell needs food so that it can keep alive and fulfil its optimum function. The intrinsic working of the human cell is an absolute marvel with actions and reactions that are very complicated and still somewhat beyond understanding. The complete life force within the cell is so fascinating and is a clear reflection of life itself. Despite how complicated the cell is, it just keeps on working, guided by some life force that does show a respect for order and logic. Sometimes we humans just don't understand the ordered function of this life. We try so hard to control or change it. We need to tune into this logically ordered life function and somehow just let it happen rather than force it to happen. We need to stop trying to change it so as to suit our scientific understanding of it.

It is beyond understanding how a cell works and what it is that controls it, let alone how many millions of these cells can work together in harmony to collectively make up an organ and allow it to do its function. Then all the organs of our body function in unison with each other to keep a body alive. What a marvel it is that an egg and sperm can join to become one cell and then multiply and grow into a complete human, which if feed and protected will live for up to 100 years or more regularly repairing and fixing itself.

The only thing the cell needs in abundance to keep alive is oxygen and food i.e. water, vitamins, minerals, energy, protein, fats and antioxidants. There may very well be other ingredients that the cell uses that we have not yet identified. One of the biggest mistakes we make is to presume we already know it all. I am sure there are a lot of things about the human body we don't know. We just don't know that we don't know it.

So if you want to keep your body alive, put alive things into it. It really is as simple as that. The majority of your food should be the same as when nature made it, alive and fresh. At least 80% of the diet should be plants, fresh and preferably locally grown. The sooner you can eat the food after it has been harvested the better it is for you, because more life force (Mauri Ora) remains in it.

Many people do struggle with growing, selecting and preparing fresh produce. It is perceived that preparing healthy food is a lot of extra work. Processed food is so much quicker, easier, and more readily available. The processing has often changed and altered the flavour, taste and texture so it is more attractive to our palate. Many people think that healthy food is more expensive than quick fast food. This is not true. Bottom line is we are very lazy when it comes to growing and preparing food. We need to be eating better food and we need to be putting in a greater effort to do that. If we put a little time into the forward planning of our meals it is very cheap to eat healthy food, it will be better on our wallets and better for our health. Good health saves money.

Basic Food Guidelines

1. Have a wide variety of vegetables, fruits, nuts, seeds and grains. Choose many different colours and textures. Strong colours indicate a strong presence of antioxidants, more power and protection for your body.

2. Once you have your fresh food items, keep them alive. Don't store them in plastic or keep them for too long before eating them. Microwaving kills the life force in foods, so don't microwave your food. Do not over cook your food. Raw plants are generally better than cooked plants.

3. The majority of your food should be plants. Animal and animal products should make up less than 20% of your food. Have a wide variety of animal products, not just a few. Most people think that chicken is a healthy food. I do not believe it is. If you enjoy eating meat make sure you have a wide variety, not just fish and chicken.

4. Find the healthy foods that you like. Don't force yourself to eat what doesn't taste good. The adventure of digestion begins in the mouth as saliva flows in anticipation of something delicious. This is the beginning of the process of breaking down food to nourish our cells.

5. Eat in season. Be adventurous in finding fresh fruits and vegetables; look at different recipe books to get ideas about what you could be eating.

6. Eat small portions and often. Have at least three good meals daily with small snacks between.

7. Choose low glycaemic foods. These are foods that have a slow energy release. They are natural foods, where as high glycaemic foods are mainly processed foods.
8. Don't over indulge, but also be aware of under eating.
9. Eat foods that don't have labels on them. This will mean they have not been processed.
10. When you can, support locally grown food suppliers. Their food will have more life in it because it is fresh.
11. When shopping at the supermarket try and get most of your items from around the outside area of the shop. This is where most of the fresh fruit and vegetable produce is found. Up and down the aisle is where most of the processed food is.
12. The most vibrant food, and therefore the best for you, is that which you have grown yourself in your own backyard.

Be thankful for your food. Appreciate its value and what it does to support the body you live in. The purpose of food is to keep you alive and healthy. Fresh food is alive. A living thing will do its job better if you communicate with it, so by choosing to resonate with your food it will assist its assimilation.

Therefore be grateful and thankful when preparing the food and thankful to the earth for producing good food for you. When giving thanks for your food, politely tell/ask the food to do its job well and keep you vibrant. That is foods job, to keep you healthy. Have a high level of expectation that your food will do a good job of keeping you well. That alone will make a big difference as to how live food will function in your body. There is a lot of scientific study now showing how thought can affect matter. Check out 'The Hidden Messages in Water' by Masaru Emoto.

Your body knows what is good for it. If you give the body a wide variety of choices and mindfully listen to it the body will tell you what it needs. Find the healthy foods that you like and eat them. Just because a food is healthy does not mean you have to like it and eat it. Enjoy the healthy foods that your body likes. In choosing to build a closer relationship with your body, be mindful of the long term effects rather than short term pleasure.

Breakfast is important, every meal is important, but because we do a lot of our healing and repair work while we sleep, the body will be low on energy when we wake. Approximately 60% of our energy consumption happens when we are sleeping. We need to re-fuel the body each time we wake. We have just had the best part of 10 hours of high energy consumption while sleeping and no food going in to replenish the energy level.

The body therefore needs a good level of nutrient rich food at the end of the day to set things up for a good sleep. With a lot of maintenance, repair and growth happening during the sleep time, it is important we have the right level of nutrients available for that function.

Nutrition at the Cellular Level

Having a good level of nutrition available at the cellular level is what keeps our body alive and well. For me there are only four main areas to this food/nutrition equation.

1. First is the quality and quantity of food.
2. How well do we digest the food? Efficiency of stomach and intestine.
3. Once absorbed into the blood, how well does the blood work at transporting the food to our cells.
4. Lastly is the metabolism. How efficient are your cells at using the food.

Food Quality and Quantity

I have covered this point at the start of this chapter. It is all very simple. If you want to keep your body alive, put alive foods into it. Find fresh alive foods that you enjoy the taste of and eat them in appropriate quantities.

A diet does not have to be fancy or a lot of hard work. A diet of fresh simple foods can still be a very healthy diet. But also be prepared to experiment with different food types. Who knows, they might taste a lot better than you thought.

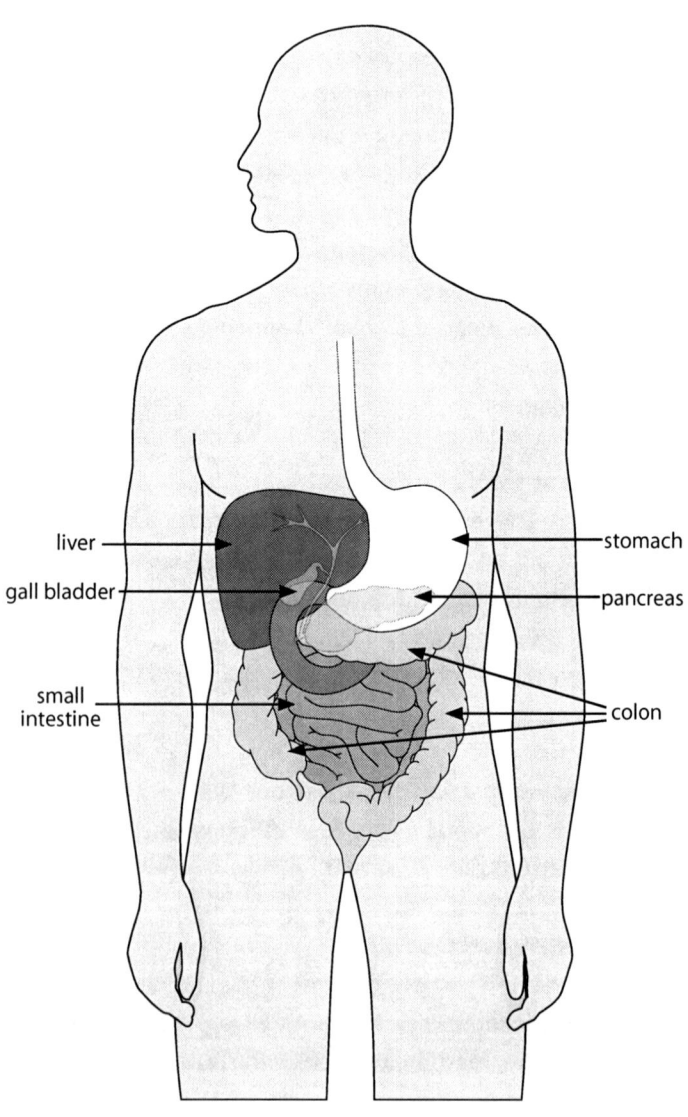

Digestion

For me this is the biggest problem we are facing in the adult human body. It is very rare to find any adult in the Western world who has very good digestion. Let me repeat that statement. It is very rare to find an adult in the Western world who has very good digestion.

In my practise I have seen for many years that the single most common problem is our poor ability to digest our food and an even poorer ability to absorb that digested food into the blood via the intestine. I do believe the underlying core health issue for most adult humans is our inability to digest the food.

Two of the biggest consumed drugs in the western world are Losec and Somac. These drugs are only ever prescribed when there are digestive tract problems. They are never used for anything else, just digestion. By the fact that they are among the heaviest used drugs, it is therefore very clear to me that one of the biggest problems we face, by number, is digestion. Most people using these drugs notice a good improvement in their symptoms. They feel much better, which therefore means taking the drug is a very good option for many thousands of people. However, if they stop using the drug, their symptoms will nearly always return. Most will have negative symptoms in their digestion within 24 hours. The medication does not fix the problem, it only masks the symptoms.

There are many people who have bad digestive track symptoms, and mostly they will do something about it. They know they have a problem because there are clear negative symptoms. There are an even larger number of people who have poor digestion but don't know it, because there are no obvious signs that their digestion is inefficient. For most adults our digestion will be poor. It gets very poor over a long period of time, starting in our childhood/teenage years. The digestive efficiency will get lower in very small incremental steps. Usually so small we don't notice.

It takes many years to get to a very low level of efficiency.

Now, one of the worst aspects of this whole digestive scenario is the fact that if we improve our diet and eat extremely well, particularly having foods that are recommended to help our digestion, I do not see any significant improvement in our over all digestive ability. The digestive system might feel better, and usually does feel better if we eat good natural alive food, but very seldom is the efficiency of digesting that food any better. So we will still have a digestive track problem but not know it. Good digestion or not, we are better off trying to digest good food than not so good food.

Every cell in our body requires food so as to do its function. Every piece of food required by our cells has to come via the digestion system. The digestion system is the port hole for life to enter your cells.

What makes the Digestion Poor?

Over the years all of us are putting things into the stomach that the stomach was not designed to deal with. The most obvious thing is processed food, which we are having in ever increasing amounts. This food has been altered, radically changed from its original state as a plant or an animal, whatever it was. Within that processing, much of the food will have had preservatives and chemicals added to it. In that processing a lot of nutrients are depleted and changed. The food was once in a living healthy state, but now when we get it in the processed form it does not have the same vitality. There is a huge amount of chemicals coming through the food chain itself right from the growing stage, and then more are usually added at the food processing, packaging and storage stage. Most of these chemicals have been tested and are apparently of 'no harm to humans' if used in the appropriate ways. One can make up ones own mind as regards the safety of chemical fertilisers, sprays, and preservatives. The intention of this book is not to rake the mud if there is nothing to be gained by doing so. I am sure everyone reading this book will already have made their own decisions as regards chemicals in the food chain. Commonsense clearly says that prudent avoidance of all chemicals is the best option.

There are a many different things that negatively interfere with our digestive system – processed foods, over cooked foods, fizzy drinks, high energy drinks, microwaved food, (check the chapter on the microwave) prescription and over the counter drugs, too much meat/protein, juice concentrates – especially orange juice, and fast foods. For some it is just the large volume of food they are having over a long period of time. Because there is so much food going in to the stomach, it does not have to be efficient.

Most of us at sometime in our lives have consumed many different types of food that have a negative effect on the stomach. Just because your digestion system feels good does not mean it is functioning efficiently. Please don't fool yourself that you are one of the lucky ones with good digestion and it is all the others that have the problem.

The Intestine

The small intestine is where we are supposed to absorb the digested food into our blood for distribution around the body. The small intestine is approximately 6 metres long. Different parts of the intestine deal with different nutrients. This is a very complex organ with a huge surface area so as to absorb all the required nutrients. However, for the purpose of this chapter I want to keep it simple. The primary function of the intestine is to transfer nutrients from the food that was digested in the stomach into the blood stream. Over many years there will be a gradual build up of poorly digested food in the small nooks and crannies of the intestine. This will cut down the area available for absorption and thus reduce the amount of nutrient arriving in the blood.

Nearly every adult will have very poor function in the intestine. This is mainly because the food in our stomach has been digested very poorly and this will clog up the intestine. Poorly digested food is devastating in this area. Too much meat and fat are also very bad for this area, along with too many highly possessed grains, i.e. wheat, rice etc.

Poor liver function is also devastating on the intestine and colon. I have covered this issue in the liver chapter. Be sure to read about the liver so as to understand the negative effect a poor liver can have on the digestion system. It promises to answer a lot of concerns you may have with your lower digestive system.

The colon is an area for further absorption of nutrients and also the area of our digestive track where we can get rid of toxins from around the body. Fibre plays a very important role here. There are two types of fibre; soluble fibre and insoluble fibre. Most of us are well aware of the insoluble fibre. It is the rough stuff we get from whole grain cereals, especially bran. This is needed in the intestine to help scrape out any lazy food particles that take lodging in all those little groves. When this fibre enters the digestive system it swells up once it has had time to react with our digestive juices. This helps it to expand in the small intestine and push into those tight spots to keep everything moving well.

The soluble fibre is quite different. We get this mainly from fruits and vegetables. Being soluble it is dissolved into our digestive juices, absorbed into the blood and then carried around the body in our circulation system. It has the ability to mop up toxins and waste products in the blood system and then take them back to the colon where they are extracted from the body. The colon is a very large dumping ground for our waste. Because most people have poor colon function it is very hard to eliminate all the waste we need to, both the waste from our food and the waste picked up by the soluble fibre.

Good healthy food is not just for feeding our bodies with the right energy, vitamins and minerals. It also provides us with some very important cleaning agents – fibre. We should have a 1:2 ratio of insoluble fibre to soluble in our diet.

Let me give a very basic explanation of the digestive system. There are three parts to it. Stomach, intestine and colon. After we have chewed our food and mixed it with saliva it is swallowed into the stomach where the acids, bacteria and enzymes break it down further. It is then released into the long thin small intestine for further digestion and absorption into the blood system. The small intestine is about 6 metres long and has a surface area equivalent to the size of a tennis court. The food particles that are still in the intestine are then moved on into the colon which starts on our right-hand side by the appendix area. The colon goes up our right side, across under the ribs and then down to the anal area. This may sound like an explanation that is shared with a five year old. I know it is a very basic description but it is very important that we see it in such a basic crude way.

I mentioned earlier the importance of eating fresh alive food. If our food is of poor quality and high in fat and animal proteins it can very quickly clog up all the fine surface area of the small intestine. High fibre diets help to keep the surface area scraped clean. There have been many leading health experts who have clearly stated their belief that 'Death starts in the colon'. This is something I have also seen repeated over and over for many years. With this understanding there is now many different solutions being offered to get the colon working better.

Many of these solutions revolve around food selections that help to clean out the intestine and colon. These may be effective in moving out the rubbish that has built up but they very seldom improve your ability to digest good nutrients out of the food. Probiotics are well used and highly recommended by many experts. These probiotics are usually supplemental bacteria that can help to break down your food for you. This will usually result in the passage of food through your body being more comfortable. We feel better in the digestive area so therefore think the products are of benefit. We assume our digestion is better.

However in most cases the efficiency of our digestion has not improved. The ability to extract nutrients from the food has usually not changed. Every cell in your body has the same DNA, whether that cell is from the skin, blood, bone, heart or even the DNA of the digestive bacteria and enzymes, they all have exactly the same DNA. The digestive enzymes and bacteria break down the food to be compatible with all your cells. Introduced probiotic break the food down but not always to be fully compatible with your cells. When one stops taking a probiotic it is not long before the digestion slips back to its former poor function. Thus problem not solved.

What is needed is Prebiotics. Prebiotics have the ability to make your own digestive enzymes and bacteria breed. You will make more of your own digestive aids in the stomach so as to break your food down more completely. This means more nutrients will be available for your cells. Food that is digested completely will help to clean out the intestine and colon and keep them functioning in a healthy state. This in turn will make it easier to absorb more nutrients into the blood for feeding the cells of your body.

Other solutions for the digestion include colon irrigation and enema use. This can be good for removing everything out of the colon area. It gives the colon a good wash-out. However, it does not necessarily make the colon work more efficiently. Most would presume that this clean out would make it more efficient in the colon but this is not always the case. The life and efficiency of the colon is totally determined by what happens in the digestive system before the colon, i.e. intestine and stomach.

If good quality alive food is put into the stomach and digested well it will help to keep the intestine and colon healthy. If the food is of poor quality and highly processed it is more likely to clog up the colon. It is important that when we ingest food it is a balanced meal consisting of carbohydrates, proteins, fats and fibre. Each food group is required by the others for complete and balanced digestion.

I mentioned earlier in this chapter that there are four main aspects about food;
1. Quality and quantity of our food
2. Digestion and absorption into our blood
3. The ability of the blood to get the food to our cells
4. Metabolism of the nutrients in our cells

I have covered the first two issues thus far. The third issue with food is to do with the ability of our blood to flow through our blood vessels. It also looks at the ability of our blood to carry our nutrients to our cells where they are needed for optimal health. Can the blood flow freely through our arteries, veins and capillaries? Is the blood quality good enough so as to carry the nutrients to our cells? The ability of the blood to carry our nutrients to our cells will mainly be covered in the kidneys chapter. The kidney function has a huge impact on our blood quality.

There are several different reasons why our blood quality will be low; however the most common reason I see for poor quality blood is poor kidney function. The ability or freedom of our blood to circulate through our blood vessels will be talked about in the chapter covering heart disease.

The fourth and final issue with food is the metabolism of our food. When people are asked to explain metabolism most will think of having a fast or slow metabolism but will not know how to explain it further than that. True metabolism is 'a measure of how efficient are your cells at using food once the food has arrived at the cell'. When the vitamins, minerals, antioxidants and energy have arrived at your cells, how good are the cells at using these nutrients? This is a very big problem for those with kidney problems but is easily fixed.

Poor metabolism at the cellular level is rather common and is very easy to fix. The simplest way to get metabolism up to speed is with a herbal tea made from sage. Put either fresh or dried sage in a cup, pour on the hot water from the kettle and then drink. It is as simple as that. Five cups of this tea is the maximum one should have at any time. If you have too much sage tea it may imbalance hormonal levels and also it will loose its effectiveness for when it is really needed.

So I have now covered the quantity and quality of food with some basic guidelines on how to get the food correct. Remember if you want to keep your body alive then put alive food items into it.

To get your blood and circulation up to scratch read the chapters covering kidney function and heart disease.

Metabolism is very easy to sharpen up with a sage tea. Now all that is left to deal with is digestion.

To get the digestion functioning at a better level it is a little more complicated. In my many years of dealing with people with poor health I have found only one thing that has the ability to improve digestive function. There are many things that can help to make the digestion feel better and that is always good for the person concerned. However we need to make it function better.

I am now left in a big dilemma. Because of company rules and regulations I am not allowed to put into print any nutritional products or supplements that I feel may be of benefit. I am allowed to make broad statements like 'vitamin C may be good for the immune system' or 'magnesium may help some people to sleep better', but I cannot mention any products or product names. I find this frustrating but these are the rules.

I have seen one particular supplement change the digestive ability for many people. It is the only thing I have found that has the ability to make our stomach produce more digestive bacteria and enzymes. But I am not allowed to mention this in a book. The easiest way to get this information to you the reader is via email. This may be a lot of extra work for me but I do feel very strongly about this area of health. I am prepared to share with you through email what is the best and only solution I have found thus far for getting the digestive system up to a good efficient level. It is a serious issue that has to be dealt with because it is the biggest health problem I see in the adult population. So please feel free to email me on the email address found at the back of this book, and I will endeavour to get this information to you as soon as I can.

In the mean time do your best to put only alive plants into your digestive system. It will make a difference to your health. Let me repeat the quote. 'What you eat and drink today will make you walk and talk tomorrow'.

CHAPTER THREE
KIDNEYS

Your kidneys are the filters - their primary job is to filter your pollution out of the blood and put it into your bladder. Poor kidney function is a huge problem from the point of view that many people are afflicted by it. Poor kidney function is a huge problem because of how much damage is done in the body and how it has such a negative effect on other organs and body functions.

There are four main ways that we get rid of pollution out of our body:
1. We breathe some out
2. We sweat through the skin
3. We pass waste through the bowel
4. We pass pollution through the kidneys and bladder

To my knowledge there is no medical test available to measure whether your kidneys can filter your pollution out of your blood into the bladder. There are many different tests that can be done to check for kidney size, infections, blood flow and urine flow, blockages, kidney stones, cancer, inflammation, etc. But there is no test to see whether they can do their primary job of filtering your pollution out of your body. Poor kidney function is a very,

very common problem, and the worst aspect is the fact that it is un-diagnosable.

The Symptoms
Common symptoms when kidneys are poor are; continual tiredness, black under the eyes, headaches, migraines, tight neck muscles, poor circulation, light-headedness, dizziness, bruising easily, heart palpitations, frequent bladder activity at night, feeling thirsty and drinking a lot of water but remaining thirsty, fluid retention as evidenced by swelling, cramping of muscles, feeling cold, deteriorating eyesight, short term memory problems, lack of energy, high blood pressure, hormonal issues, pre-menstrual problems, infertility problems, pregnancy problems, poor learning ability, high cholesterol, low iron and B vitamins, sugar (high glycaemic) cravings, constipation, weight increase. The list is long.

Many diagnosed/labelled diseases are the result of poor kidneys. Low metabolism, migraines, poor lungs, low immune system, frequent infections in the lung throat region and a general long term unwellness are all very common when the kidney function is poor. If the body cannot clean itself many problems will arise.

How Does it Work?
When we drink most of the fluid is absorbed into the blood via the transverse colon. The fluid travels through the stomach, small intestine and then colon. The brain computer knows when the cells are thirsty and so instructs the transverse colon to suck out the amount of fluid required. The more dehydrated the cells are the more fluid is required. The greater the fluid removed from the colon area, the drier the food (faecal matter) will be, resulting in probable constipation.

The renal glands are the main controllers of how much fluid is absorbed at the cellular level. These glands are closely connected with the kidneys and the kidney function. If kidney function is low it is most likely that the renal gland function will also be low. This will normally result in the cells of the body being very de-hydrated.

The main cells to de-hydrate are brain cells and muscle cells. De-hydrated muscles are tight and less pliable. Most people will suffer tight neck shoulder muscles and possibly be prone to leg muscle cramps at night. De-hydration also affects the muscle tissue that controls bowel motion. This further adds to the constipation problem. Our muscles must be fully hydrated.

Headaches

De-hydrated brain cells create headaches and in severe cases migraines and vision problems. Most headaches are closely associated with de-hydration. At this point most people are feeling constantly thirsty and drink copious amounts of water, yet still feel de-hydrated and have no improvement of health symptoms. Drinking more is not the solution. Just because we drink a lot of water does not mean our cells are getting that fluid. What really matters is whether the fluid gets into our cells. Are our cells capable of absorbing the correct amount of fluid?

Skin

This de-hydration starts to affect our skin. Most people with poor kidneys will have poor skin, more prone to pimples, dark under the eyes, and bags under the eyes. Also because the blood has not been filtered clean it is most likely some will experience skin rash, boils and/or skin infections. Poor blood results in poor skin colour. Most will be constantly pale in the face, but when they exercise they will become very flushed in the face area.

When kidney function is poor too much of your own pollution is left in your blood. This will have a very negative effect on your blood's ability to do its job correctly. Basically your blood is a transport system. It just carries things around the body. It takes good things into your cells, i.e. food, water, oxygen, and then takes the rubbish out to the kidneys, liver, lungs, colon and skin where it can be extracted from the body.

Many elderly people suffer from skin problems on the lower leg and feet area. It is very common for a small scratch on the leg/foot area to end up as a large ulcer. The poor blood supply which is low in nutrient and high in pollution make it very hard for healing to take place. It is then easier for infections to get rooted in the skin. To compound these issues is the fact that as we age it is common to suffer from poor circulation –that is the ability for the blood to flow through our arteries, capillaries and veins. So there is a poor supply of blood and the blood that does get there is of poor quality. It is therefore very hard to heal. This can affect all skin areas but especially the arms, hands, legs and feet.

Oxygen

Poor blood quality means a lower level of oxygen in the body. This results in a person feeling cold and always having cold hands and feet. When we stand too quickly we may experience light-headedness, dizziness. Many have to move slowly and hold for balance. Breathlessness and hypo-ventilating is because of a lack of oxygen in the blood. Many times the people will experience the heart racing. This is usually just the heart, under instructions from the brain, pumping more blood through the lungs hoping to get more oxygen in to the blood. But because the blood is polluted due to poor kidney function, it will not be able to carry the required amount of oxygen.

Lungs

There is a very strong connection between the kidneys and the lungs. If the kidneys are not getting rid of the rubbish, it will many times pollute the lungs. Most people with serious/chronic lung problems will nearly always have poor kidneys. The poor kidneys are the core reason for the poor lungs. On-going lung infections will require antibiotic medication. This will usually clear the infection but put further pressure on already low kidneys, which continue to give us bad blood which in turn makes us vulnerable to further infection, then more antibiotic. It is just an on-going vicious cycle. How often do we see this in the people we know and love, especially the young and the elderly.

There are a lot of young children who continually suffer from lung infections. Many of these young ones do have very poor lungs but they do not have lung infections. They have high mucus levels and symptoms that are very similar to asthma. The asthma medications sometimes bring a little relief, but many times don't. It is very likely that they have on-going poor kidney function. The poor kidney function will junk-up the lungs.

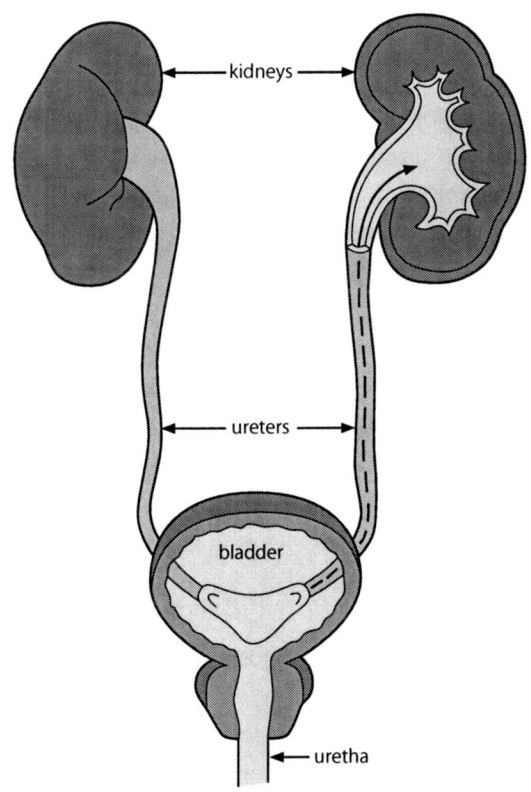

Fluid Retention

When we get de-hydrated we are likely to suffer headaches. When we get severely de-hydrated we are likely to suffer migraines. For women the next common stage is fluid retention. Because the body is de-hydrated it will try and retain fluid in the fluid system – mainly the lymphatic system and then around our cells but not in the cell. We see many people very puffed up around the lower leg/foot area and also heavily around the mid-torso area. Many get diagnosed with fluid around the heart and lung area. It becomes a very confusing and conflicting situation. Retaining large amounts of fluid but at the same time feeling very de-hydrated. Always thirsty, so drinking plenty, but having frequent bladder activity to get rid of all that water that has been consumed. People taking medication to help remove excess fluid and yet at the cellular level they are already very de-hydrated.

Bladder

Frequent urination at night time will have more to do with poor kidney function than prostrate or bladder functions. How this works is the body does know it is polluted with too much of its own pollution and knows that this type of pollution can only be removed via the kidney/bladder. So as soon as there is enough fluid in the bladder to trigger urination, the body will clearly tell you to go to the toilet. How often are we busting to go to the toilet and have to get there ASAP but when we do there is only a small dribble? Maybe only half a cup. This is just the body urgently trying to get rid of some pollution. Just clearing a small amount is better than clearing none at all. Also be aware that most bladder infections are the result of poor kidney function.

Tiredness

The single most common symptom when kidneys are poor is tiredness. Always feeling tired regardless of the amount of sleep we have had. And sometimes even when we can get extra sleep we feel more tired. Along with this tiredness we will feel a lack of strength and energy. After exercising we will have a slower recovery period than what would be normal. It is hard to get stimulated both physically and mentally. You know what you need to do but just cannot do it.

Because the blood quality is low it has a poor ability to hold energy and nutrients. Therefore most people with low kidneys have a tendency for high energy foods, such as sweets, chocolate and high glycaemic foods. They need energy instantly. Quality energy and nutrients from low glycaemic food is too slowly released for the body's urgent needs. These cravings can be very similar to a diabetic situation. A lot of people with kidney function problems show very clear diabetic symptoms, yet do not have diabetes.

The poor blood quality in our bodies will commonly show up that we are low in iron. Many people have blood tests to check their iron and find they are low. They then take the obvious step of taking an iron supplement. But why don't we ask the obvious question, "why are we deficient of iron?" Poor kidney function is not the only reason for being low in iron but it is a common contributing factor.

Muscle

I mentioned how the muscles get very dry and tight. The next step for a lot of people is to then get a massage. This can help take some tension out of the muscle. How many times have we had a massage that has really hurt? The masseuse will frequently tell us that we are very tight around the neck and shoulder area and the massage hurts. We may feel a good benefit from the massage for 3–4 days but are then back to square one. This is because the masseuse is massaging dry tough muscle/meat. I don't mean to put any massage people out of business, but if we got our kidneys and renal glands functioning better so as to correct the hydration, we would get a better and longer lasting result from our massages. We would not require frequent massages and the massage we do have will be more about pleasure than pain.

Brain

With poor kidney function many people start to notice short term memory problems. If the kidney function happened to dropped low about 4 months back, you will find that over the last 3 months the memory for every day things will be getting very poor. If eye sight is poor the deterioration and degeneration in this area will also be accelerated.

There can also be a big negative impact on our learning ability. Brain function will get low because of the high pollution level in our blood. Our ability to learn and recall what we have learnt is thus very poor. Many children I see with learning difficulties and concentration problems have poor kidneys. Bad behaviour problems then come along.

Let me expand on this.

For me there are three main measures for intellectual ability,
1.   What am I capable of intellectually?
2.   What have I actually learnt?
3.   What do my teachers/parents think I've learnt?

If there is a big deficit between what I have actually learnt and what I am capable of learning, the subconscious mind will pick up on this and get very frustrated. This will then get manifested as frustrated and confused behaviour. It will be hard to concentrate. There is a deep down internal frustration about the whole learning process.

If I am learning up to my capabilities but am unable to regurgitate that information to the teacher/parent so as to prove that I have learnt the said knowledge, over time there will be even greater frustration. This will most times show up as ADD, ADHD, and /or other very disturbing behavioural problems. Deep down the brain is saying "I know all this stuff but I can't prove it and they all think I'm dumb so what's the point of trying." The first stage of this is just the inability to concentrate and then slowly becoming the class clown. What's the point of trying to learn if they all think I'm dumb?

Blood Pressure

There are many people I have seen with high blood pressure who have poor kidneys. The heart rate is usually higher than it otherwise would be and there is often an elevation of the cholesterol. There is more about cholesterol and heart disease in a later chapter.

Pregnancy

One of the most emotionally difficult health issues is infertility. This is a huge problem, sometimes creating very tense relationship situations. Poor kidney function is the single most common reason I see why a woman cannot fall pregnant. The poor blood quality has a very detrimental effect in the ovary area, making it very hard for the ovaries to produce eggs. Sometimes the egg is produced but is not healthy enough to be able to be fertilised. When the kidney function is at a very low level for more than one year it is quite normal for the female reproductive system to close down.

Even if a woman can fall pregnant with poor kidneys, it is sometimes hard to stay pregnant. The high level of pollution in her body makes it a very undesirable place for foetal development. Miscarriages are very common at this point. If the pregnancy does go to full time it will nearly always be very difficult, with high fluid retention, possible toxaemia and a probable early delivery.

A woman's menstruation period is much more difficult when she has poor kidney function. High premenstrual tension and longer bleeds are very common. Menstruation becomes rather spasmodic and some can go long periods without menstruating.

Metabolism

The meaning of metabolism for me is 'how efficient are your cells at using the food once it gets into the cells'. When the nutrients and energy get into a cell it is then available for the cell to use so as to do its function, whether it be a brain cell, heart cell, or any cell of your body. True metabolism is a measure of how efficient your cells are at using those nutrients.

When the body is polluted because of bad kidney function, it will nearly always have a very bad metabolic rate. This effectively cuts down the nutrient level in the cell. The cell will then not be able to perform at optimal levels. The lower the kidneys are the lower the metabolism will be. The greatest effect is in the brain cell area. This usually has a very negative influence on how well our brain cells recall information, our learning ability, and mental motivation. Short term memory loss will be poorer than long term memory loss.

Solution

There are several different solutions when your kidneys are functioning poorly. The most common one I recommend is a simple parsley tea. Get a small sprig of fresh parsley and put it in a cup. Boil the kettle and pour the water into the cup. If you do know or suspect that your kidney function is poor then you need to have 2-3 cups of this parsley tea each day for 3 days, then cut it back to one cup daily for at least 3 weeks. In most cases this will get the kidneys functioning better.

Do not microwave this tea. If it has been microwaved it will not work. The tea can be drunk hot, warm or cold. The most important thing is to have the boiling water from the kettle poured over the herb. You can leave it until it is cold to drink if you wish. It can then be put in a drink bottle and topped up with fresh water so as to be consumed throughout the day. A fresh brew should be made each day.

This does not always correct the hydration at the cell level, so what I recommend is to add a small piece of rosemary to that parsley tea. The rosemary is good for stimulating some life into the renal glands, so as to correct the hydration. This rosemary can be fresh or dried. Just put a small amount of the herb into the cup with the parsley for up to 3 days, but no longer. If you enjoy the rosemary tea it is all alright to have it on an occasional basis – 1-2 cups weekly. Typically rosemary is used as an additive to meat dishes. It helps to tenderise the meat. If your meat/muscle is tight, sore or injured then have 2-3 cups of rosemary tea. It can help in the recovery.

As mentioned above, the metabolism of the body at the cell level will nearly always be low if your kidneys are functioning poorly. To correct this put a small amount of sage into the parsley/rosemary tea. Do this for three days only. It is the best simple way I know of stimulating the metabolism. The sage can be fresh or dried. Use two leaves if fresh or ½ teaspoon if dried. The sage is also great for helping correct the hormonal function in the body.

So there are three herbs – parsley, rosemary and sage - in the same cup or teapot for three days only, then after the three days continue with just the parsley for a few weeks. It is that simple. There are several other things you can do to improve kidney function, but this is the best simple way I've seen.

Some other options include nettle tea and dandelion leaf tincture. There are many more solutions that are recommended from lots of publications but I have not seen any of these working well on a regular basis. Cranberry juice or cranberry extract are many times recommended when there are kidney and bladder problems, but from what I have seen cranberry is mainly for repairing the kidney/bladder area. The cranberry is not so good at turning the organ function on. The parsley turns it on so the cranberry can then help with the repair. If it is not turned on it cannot be repaired.

Now that the kidneys are working better there will be better blood carrying more nutrients to all parts of the body, so repair can be achieved at the cell level everywhere. Good quality nutrients at the cellular level in the body are what do the real repair. This is what quality food is for --- on-going optimum health for many years.

How Much Water?

There is a lot of information in the public arena saying we need to drink 8-10 glasses of water each day. I do not always agree with this. Just because we are drinking a lot of water does not mean the cells are getting it. Kidney and renal gland function are the main controllers of hydration at the cellular level. If you are always drinking too much it may help you to feel full in the stomach and therefore stop you eating as much as you should. The amount of water we consume can and will vary from one person to another and from day to day. Don't count your glasses. Drink when the body tells you to. On hot days you might need more than on cold days. If you are eating a quality diet of fresh fruit and vegetables you will be consuming 4-5 cups of water each day from that food. Lots of water going through the body does not get rid of the toxins and pollutants. It is efficient kidneys, liver and colon that are the main filters of this rubbish from our body.

I hope this has enlightened you on a few issues relating to kidney problems. It is easy to see how important good kidney function is and also how many everyday health problems can be traced back to poor kidney function. Remember that at this point there is no simple test you can get done at your doctor that can tell you whether your kidneys are capable of filtering your rubbish out of your body. Do everything you need to do to keep your kidneys happy. Your body will thank you for it.

LIVER

When you analyse the human body as one functional object, it is easy to come to the conclusion that the liver is the centre of the body. Everything revolves around the liver and the liver function has a huge influence over many parts of the body and sometimes a very complete controlling influence. In particular the digestive system. The liver is the most multi-tasked part of our body and does many different jobs.

The acidity level in our body is totally controlled by the liver. Stomach acid travels into the intestine with digested foods. Bile is produced in the liver, stored in the gallbladder, and then when it is needed it is released into the small intestine via the bile duct so as to neutralize the stomach acids as they travel into the intestine with the digested food.

These days there is a greater awareness of the importance of a correct pH level in the body. Most people try to correct their pH with different food options. More and more people are getting onto alkaline foods to help with health issues. This is all very good but from my experience nearly all acid in your body is controlled by the liver function, not the foods we eat.

If liver function is low, there will not be enough bile produced so as to neutralize those stomach acids when they enter the small intestine. Too much of the stomach acid that enters the intestinal tract will then be absorbed into the blood. This acid is then carried around the body and can have a very negative effect on cell tissues. The stomach is supposed to be acidic. This acidity plays an important role in breaking down our food. The acid cannot get absorbed through the stomach lining into our blood. Acidity only becomes a problem once the acids get into the intestine.

Some of the more common functions of the liver include; detoxifying the blood, production and maintenance of blood cells, quality of skin, acidity regulation, it technically is a gland so has a big influence over other glands, emotional centre, metabolism of fats and proteins, mineral storage, especially iron and folates, plus many more important functions. There is no one liver function test that can check for all the functions that the liver does. Ideally there should be a number of different tests for all the different things the liver does.

When the liver function is poor some of the common symptoms are; excess wind and bloating, sensitivity to food, food shooting through the system too quickly, loss of appetite, eating small meals often, and many other issues mainly revolving around food. Because the acids from the stomach are not being neutralized when they enter the intestine they get absorbed into our blood and carried throughout our body. This usually has a direct connection with eczema problems and similar skin issues such as cirrhosis of the skin. This acidity also has a very detrimental effect on our joints. More on that issue later when we cover arthritis problems.

The high acidity level fogs up the brain. People will feel as if they have a cloud in their brain all the time. Memory recall and decision making are usually very slow. Even while in a conversation people find they very quickly run out of words, or lose their thinking process.

The acidity level creates a lot of mucus, especially in the sinus areas and in the upper lung and throat area. And then to add fuel to that problem, when we eat dairy foods, particularly milk, cheese and ice-cream, (yoghurt generally doesn't fall in to this category) we are likely to produce more mucus. When we are

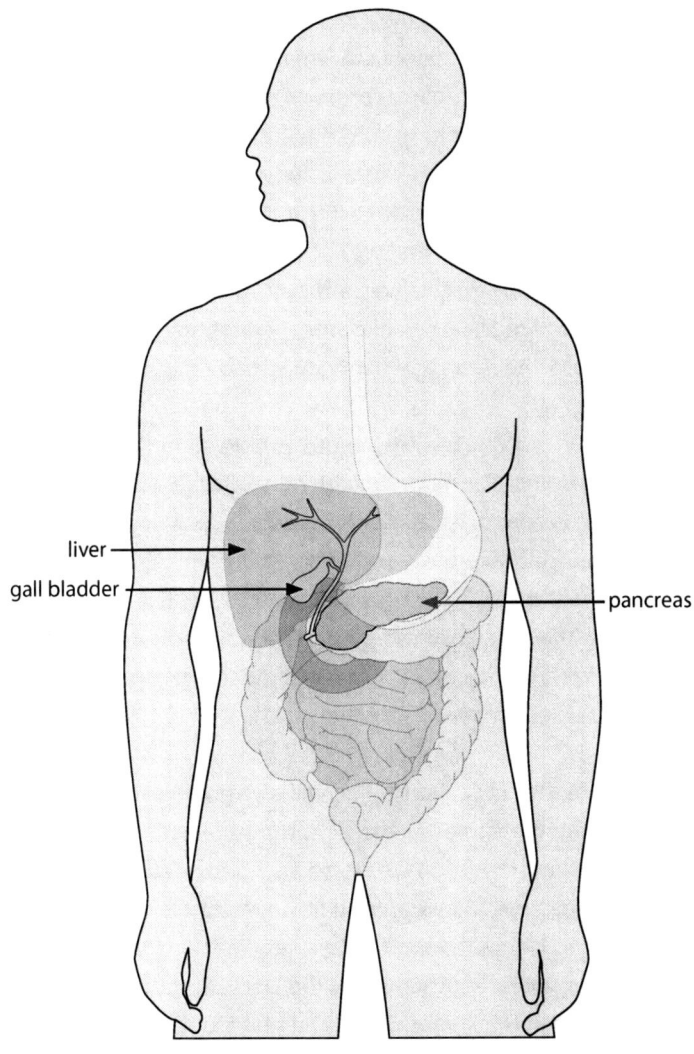

liver

gall bladder

pancreas

acidic and having reasonable quantities of those foods we are going to see a lot more mucus. Other foods that help to create a negative situation when the liver is low are any animal products, all meats including chicken, fish and shell fish. When the liver is low it doesn't like you eating things that are animal, with the exception of good yoghurt and eggs. All other animal foods particularly in large quantities tend to be hard on the liver. The problem with these foods is the fats and proteins.

The liver has to deal with the processing of meats, both fats and proteins, and it finds it very hard when it is in a low state. As you can imagine when any part or organ of the body isn't functioning well, then it is harder for it to do its job. So if your liver is low, and you know it is low, you are better off being somewhat vegetarian, having foods that are mainly plant-based. Going back to that basic diet, what we should be having is at least 80% plant. Particularly for the liver, it is best to eat alive fresh plants that are raw. Fruits, vegetables, nuts, grains, and seeds. Plants that still look the same as when nature made them.

The acidity can create very serious problems in the intestine, colon area. Heart-burn, re-flux, bloating, irritable bowel, leaky gut, polyps, celiac disease, gluten sensitivity, lactose intolerance, diarrhoea, food allergies, and many more. In most instances your GP will prescribe a common medication like Losec. This is one of the most commonly prescribed medications in the western world today, which proves to me that poor digestion is our single biggest health problem.

Most times the Losec medication will give great results, and the patient does feel fantastic, the symptoms are gone. Life is more enjoyable and they don't have to be concerned about what food they can eat and what food to stay clear of. But as soon as people stop taking the medication, very quickly the symptoms are all back again. In other words the Losec is not getting rid of the problem. It is just masking it. The real problem is not fixed.

We now have two main problems. Firstly the liver function, which in turn creates the acidity problems, and secondly a major digestion problem. The digestive system is covered in detail in the food chapter. However it is worth mentioning here that many people are aware of this acidity problem and try to rectify it with food selection. They identify which foods are acid forming and which are alkaline. Now, the stomach is supposed to be acid, so if you put too much alkaline food and drink into the stomach it may start to produce even more acid so as to keep the acid balance correct. Nearly all of the alkaline/acid balance in the body is controlled by the liver – not food. So be careful not to have too much alkaline food, it may make your body more acidic.

It is the production of bile in the liver which is then mixed with our food in the small intestine that controls acid throughout the body. We have got to be careful we do not over consume the alkaline food and drink.

A large number of people have gall-bladder problems and have the gall-bladder removed – a relatively simple operation these days. The problem then being even if you get your liver going well you don't have a storage facility for that bile. The bile is stored in the gall-bladder ready to be used as the food is released from the stomach into the intestine. The gall-bladder lets a bit of the bile down the bile duct to neutralise the stomach acids. Having no gall-bladder is going to make the acidity regulation a little bit harder, which can lead to big problems in this area long term. Short term, removal of the gall-bladder can bring in a high level of relief for the patient, but it still has not got to the root cause of why is the problem there in the first place. Why was the gall-bladder so poor that it needed to be removed? Can you now start to get a clearer understanding why the colon cancers and serious digestive tract problems are so prevalent these days, and usually have a lot to do with the liver?

CHAPTER 4

When you look at the liver in terms of its core functions, one of its functions is a detoxifying centre dealing with toxins and chemicals etc. When there is such a huge increase of chemicals going into our bodies compared to what it was a few decades ago, the liver is on overload dealing with all the toxins that we eat, drink, breathe, and put on our bodies. The liver has got a huge amount of work to do dealing with the everyday pollutants that we do put in our bodies.

The liver has to deal with animal fats. Some people are eating large amounts of animal – meat and dairy. One the most consumed animals that people are having now is chicken, in large amounts. We have been told for a few decades now that white meat is healthy and red meat is not. Chicken is regarded as a healthy meat. I have different thoughts. Of all the foods we eat, chicken is one of the only common foods that never have direct contact with the sun. All other foods we eat are either a direct result of photosynthesis or are regularly exposed to the sun, which is the source of all food energy.

We need to get away from the "chicken is healthy scenario" and think more of where did that meat come from and how has it been produced.

Normally speaking any animal that is grass fed, outdoors, has lean meat that is a healthier product compared with some of the meat that has been raised in grain fed cattle lots. Animals that are allowed to graze pasture produce meat that is much healthier and higher in omega 3 fatty acids.

However, we need to keep in mind that all of this meat /animal produce should make up a very small portion of our diet. We should be eating mainly plants. So therefore what meats we eat shouldn't be such a big issue. We need to have small portions of a wide variety of meats. It shouldn't be such a big issue about what meat you have. Just don't eat large amounts of any meat.

The liver is the emotional centre of a body. If negative emotions are going to be attached to a body, they will nearly always attach to the liver. We all have to deal with negative emotional issues from time to time in our lives, particularly with deaths and relationship problems.

Negative emotional attachments are a fairly common reason why the liver will get low in function. When there is a sudden emotional happening in our life it will usually sink into the liver. If it doesn't detach after a few days or a week, it will stay attached to the liver and then the physical function of the liver gets slowly worn down by this attachment. A lot of people are somewhat aware of that, they can still feel that negative emotion in their lives, so they do lots of talking and sharing and counselling but very rarely does that detach all that emotional attachment. Emotional things are happenings; they are not solid things like a food or chemical. It is a happening. When a happening clings on to a liver it becomes like a solid object, therefore it has to be dealt with from a physical point of view, not from a happening or a sharing/talking point of view. All the talking in the world will usually not get rid of that emotional attachment.

I regularly see four levels of emotion in a human body.
1. Emotional levels pretty good. Everything is OK.
2. Shitty, bitchy, snappy emotions. What I am talking about here is when people are at this level (shitty liver?) they know it and they can't stop it. They find they flip their lid regularly and just can't stop it. This is usually because a negative emotional happening has stayed attached to the liver.
3. Next level is more of the tearful emotions where it doesn't take much for them to trigger the waterworks. Very tearful about small things.
4. The next level down is what I would term more closed off or singular emotions. Where a person is living in a glass cocoon and they just can't get out to connect with people

on an emotional level, and people are not allowed to get in to connect with them. The lower that level gets, usually the stronger that person appears to be to the outside world. A lot of people would see this person as strong, singular with strength. They can still be a very caring loving person but it is just so hard for them to allow themselves to be attached to others on an emotional, love level and for others to be attached to them. They have always got this barrier up. A lot of people looking in will see them as being strong whereas in reality they are very closed in, closed off emotionally. Most people in this zone hate being in this zone, but just cannot break free. They become somewhat afraid or scared about connecting with people.

Having any negative emotion attached to the liver will nearly always make the liver less efficient in its function. It shows up with those common symptoms of a low liver; not really wanting to eat much, only eat now and then, grazing, the acidity, the reflux, the reactions to food.

This starts to explain how emotions and liver function and food are so directly connected. A lot of people with emotional problems have food related issues. They may find themselves using food for comfort, or get that nauseous horrible feeling in the tummy when there are emotional happenings going on. There is a very strong correlation between food, stomach, liver, and emotions. They are all so closely tied together.

Solution

There are some very simple things we all can do to help our liver function at a good level. The simplest thing I know that works nearly every time is ginger tea. The way to make this is with simple fresh root ginger. Slice a couple of thin slices of root ginger into a cup or tea pot. Boil the kettle and then pour the water in, then drink it when it is cool enough for you. It can be left until it is cold or put into a drink bottle so as to be consumed throughout the day. Do not microwave this tea or put it with anything that has been microwaved. The microwave will kill off any benefits immediately. When we first start with this ginger tea it is usually safe to have 2-3 cups a day for up to one week then cut it back to one daily. If pregnant or breast feeding do not exceed one cup daily. The only form of ginger I recommend is the fresh root, not tea bags or powdered ginger.

Milk thistle in a supplemental form is also very good for improving liver function. The best solution I know for poor liver function is dandelion root extract in a tincture/liquid form. This is excellent for stimulating the liver into life. This dandelion should only be taken for up to 10 days. However, the ginger tea is generally safe to continue with long term. If you have any of the common symptoms I mentioned in regard to poor liver function then I suggest you give the root ginger a try. Even if you do not normally like ginger, I am sure you will like this tea. When root ginger is used as a tea the taste will be very different than having ginger in your food. Most people find this tea very nice and surprisingly refreshing.

There are many liver detox products, supplements and dietary options on the market which are usually very good at detoxing your liver. But there is one very clear issue with most of them. The majority of these regimes will detox the liver but more often than not they will not turn the liver on. There is a big difference between cleaning something out and turning something on. Just because it has been cleaned out does not mean it has been turned on. Some of the detox programmes can be rather harsh on the liver. Side affects will clearly show the liver is being detoxed but do we know whether the liver has been turned on. What I believe works best is turning the liver on with some of the simple solutions mentioned and then in its own time the liver will choose when to detoxify. The whole body does know when the best time to detox is. We just need to give it all the required tools and the right environment so then the body will make the decision of when to start this detox. The body will also choose what level of detox it can handle. Some of the detox programmes can be too forced and too harsh for the body to handle. The ginger tea is very good at stimulating the liver into better life and then the liver will know what to do about a detox. The liver knows best when it can handle a detox, so let it choose, don't force it. When we are detoxifying it is best to be eating a diet high in raw plants. If the liver is low and trying to improve in function it does not want you to eat any animal products. Go vegetarian for 2-3 weeks. This will be of an enormous benefit as to how the liver feels. And having small frequent meals often helps.

Look closely at the chapters on Joints & Arthritis and Diabetes to see how the liver is the main controller of these health problems. Also in the chapter on Emotional v Mental I have expanded on some of the issues I bought up earlier in relation to emotional problems. Many of the chronic degenerative diseases we are facing in society are very directly connected to our poor liver function. Because the liver is the chemical detox centre of our body, it is worth while having ginger tea on a semi-regular basis to protect us from all the daily toxins we are exposed to. If you are in an environment where there is continual high exposure to chemicals then I would recommend that you have a daily drink of pineapple juice or eat a small amount of pineapple. Pineapple will not detox chemicals already settled in the body, but it does have the ability to stop most chemicals settling in your tissues. It is a very simple solution that can protect your body from serious problems later in life. There are many work place environments where chemical exposure is very bad but the three worst common occupations I see are car panel beaters, hair and beauty therapists and interior painters. These three examples are very common occupations where the worker is breathing in a small amount of chemical with every breath while they are at work. If you are in a work place situation where chemicals are used then please get into the practice of pineapple and ginger to protect your liver and your life. It is so good when a common food source, which is simple and cheap, is also the medicine/ insurance policy that you need to protect you against what could be a very serious health problem.

The liver technically is a gland. It is not the most important gland, but it is the biggest and it does have a large controlling affect over other glands especially the thyroid gland. If you do have a thyroid problem it will be worth while looking at the liver function as a means to help and support your thyroid. If it is chronic reflux you suffer then look directly to your liver. Eczema skin problems are usually a very direct result of the liver function being poor. If you try to fix the skin without addressing the internal problems of the liver then it maybe an up hill battle. Once you get the internals working better it is more likely that you will get the external problems improving when you use the correct skin care products. A person with acidity problems will normally have dry cracking skin with scalp problems. Dermatitis usually has acidity as the base problem.

I hope you can come to the realisation that what I have mentioned thus far about the liver is enough for you to see that it really is the centre of your body. Look after your liver well and give it the care and attention and love it deserves, because it spends all of its life looking after you. The liver is the emotional centre of the body so give it a regular feed of happy fun loving emotions.

CHAPTER FIVE
DIABETES

I need to quickly touch on this problem because it is such a fast growing problem in the western world and yet it is so easy to avoid and also very easy to control in most cases. This is a bold statement that I have just made but I do believe it, based on the evidence I have seen over many years. In most cases diabetes can be traced back to poor lifestyle choices combined with a poor functioning liver.

From my observation the main reason people are developing diabetes is very poor digestion combined with a very poor liver, over a long period of time. The liver does have a very big influence over the pancreas. A low liver will make it much harder for the pancreas to do its job well. However, having poor digestive ability will put the greatest pressure on the pancreas. I mentioned early in the chapter on food that most adults have very poor digestion. When our digestion is poor we don't just become inefficient in our ability to get nutrients from our food, we also digest and absorb that nutrient into our blood stream in an unbalanced form. Simple carbohydrates are relatively easy to absorb into our blood via the small intestine compared with all other nutrients, vitamins, minerals, proteins, fats and fibre. So therefore, when our digestion is poor, what arrives in the blood is a very high level of sugars compared with minerals, vitamins, and proteins. It is this high sugar level that puts extra stress on the pancreas. The primary function of the pancreas is to produce insulin which in turn is used for the control of sugars/energy in the blood. A high ratio of sugar in the blood creates extra work for the pancreas. When this goes on day after day for many months and years the pancreas gets either burnt out or continually over produces insulin. Thus in many cases medical intervention is required.

This may sound like an over simplified view of diabetes and even somewhat crude, but that is how I see it. Poor digestion over a long period of time creates a perfect environment for diabetes. The main reason for the poor digestion is the poor food selections we make. Then we get into the typical sugar craving situation with spiking and then hitting very low levels of blood sugar levels. This makes us want to eat more quick-fix, high energy food which just further fuels the problem. It is much quicker to digest highly processed food (high glycaemic) than unprocessed (low glycaemic) natural foods.

Highly processed food has simple carbohydrates that can be very easily digested and absorbed onto the blood which will quickly satisfy our sugar cravings. Studies have shown the benefits of chromium in helping control diabetes. The initial problem arises because of the gross imbalance of nutrients arriving in the blood, too much sugar compared with all other nutrients especially chromium. It is not necessarily a lack of chromium, but it is a low level of chromium compared with carbohydrates. The over all ratios of nutrients in the blood stream and at the cell level are more important than the total quantity. What is on the plate and what goes in the mouth is not important compared with what is in the cell. If food quality is not good on the plate then you can be sure it won't be good at the cell. However just because it is quality food on the plate does not guarantee it will be good at the cellular level. Poor food going in is the number one reason our digestion gets poor. Poor digestion is the number one reason the nutrient is poor and imbalanced at the cellular level. The ratio of nutrients at the cell level is critical for good health in all organs and systems in the body, but the most crucial area for nutrient ratio is the diabetes situation.

Because most people have poor digestion, most will also be undernourished at the cellular level which inturn will be diagnosed by the brain as "I'm hungry". This will continually tell us to eat frequently some quick fix food which also helps to build towards this diabetic situation.

When the diabetes situation gets very serious there are nearly always circulation problems that arise. If you read the chapters on liver and kidneys you will see that in both cases, especially poor kidneys, there are always negative issues for circulation. The main issue there is the quality of the blood rather than the inability of the blood to get through the blood vessels. You need to understand those two chapters clearly to get a better understanding of diabetes. When I talked about circulation you will see that there are two main aspects to circulation; one is the ability of the blood to flow through the blood vessels and the second is the quality of the blood itself. Circulation is usually below par before diabetes becomes a problem and then is further damaged by the diabetes. It is fare to say that diabetes is initially the result of some other problem, but then it becomes a problem on its own.

The most common form of diabetes is Type 2. This has been labelled mainly a lifestyle disease and I now hope that you can see how true this is. With a clear understanding of the kidney, liver, digestion and circulation areas it is easy to see how we could do a better job of controlling and even avoiding Type 2 diabetes altogether. Type 1 diabetes is linked more with genetic make-up so is therefore presumed to be harder to avoid. In my view, whether there is a genetic connection or not is somewhat irrelevant. Even if there is a genetic susceptibility, it will nearly always take something to trigger that genetic weakness, and that will usually be connected with nutrient imbalance at the cellular level. There are many human health problems that can be traced to some genetic disposition but I do feel strongly that it will nearly always take something within your own cellular environment to trigger that genetic weakness so as to produce the disease symptoms. These triggers can be many and varied but one common factor in many cases will be the poor level of nutrition at the cell level.

When kidney function is poor over a long period we will usually produce symptoms that are in line with diabetes; low in energy, sugar cravings, continually thirsty, and poor circulation especially in the hands and feet. Yet there is no diabetes. Once diabetes has been clearly diagnosed there has usually already been a long period of poor function somewhere in the body that we have not noticed or have noticed and just chosen to ignore it. A very common and clear case in point is overweight and obesity.

So what are the solutions for diabetic people? There are several things one can do to help control diabetes and they are also the same things one should do to avoid diabetes. The best solution will result in better control of the problem but more importantly for most there will be a very big improvement in overall health, more energy with increased physical and mental vitality.

We need to ensure the kidneys and liver are functioning well. Please read the chapters on kidneys and liver so as to understand their important function and get them functioning well. The biggest solution revolves around getting the digestion operating at a very efficient level. Check that out in the food chapter. For those who are suffering circulation problems because of diabetes it is very important to consume good quantities of a quality omega 3 oil. This can be fish oils or plant oils such as flax seed. There are many different oils on the market to choose from but do your best to get oil that has been manufactured to the highest standard and then make sure you take enough of it. I have covered this in depth in the chapter on heart disease and circulation.

In addition there are two things that can be fantastic for anyone with diabetes. Firstly is a chromium supplement. Get a good chromium supplement from your health store but be careful not to over dose as this can be a little hard on the kidneys. Take it at the recommended dose rate. Secondly try and get yourself some dandelion root extract in a tincture/liquid form. This is the most powerful thing I have seen for improving the liver and pancreas. Take as recommended for up to two weeks. Thereafter it can be used for one week each month for those who have a poor pancreas. There are many other nutritional and herbal things that can be tried for diabetes but I will only recommend those things that I have clearly seen give a significant improvement in a person's health.

As we all know food plays a very important roll in all diabetic situations. The most basic of rules for any diabetic is to eat often, and eat foods that are still alive. Eat foods that still look the same as when nature made them and these foods should be predominately plants. Consume a wide variety of plants that have not been processed, and that are still raw. Don't over cook or kill them in a microwave. Look for the glycaemic index, low is the best.

I do hope this has given a clear and yet simple picture of what is usually a very complicated health problem. If you can clearly understand the connection between the digestive system and the liver and then take into account the possibilities of poor kidney function for some, it should be easy to see that in most cases diabetes is the end result of having some other problem somewhere else in the body. Then when we get diabetes we all know that it will usually start to create even more health problems later in life, particularly circulation problems.

So please don't be surprised at the simple way I have pictured diabetes, instead listen to the logical commonsense. For most of us who do not have diabetes, there is nothing specific we need to do to avoid getting diabetes. No, all we have to do is the simple correct things for keeping the whole body well and then as a side affect of that we should avoid diabetes. Don't be so concerned about diabetes. Be more concerned about achieving overall good health. Avoiding diabetes will be the result of achieving good health.

CHAPTER SIX
WEIGHT CONTROL

What a very confusing issue for so many of us. Let's start with the most common basic belief about excess weight. Most people in society presume that if someone is over weight they are obviously eating too much and are physically very lazy. If this were true then all we would have to do is eat less and get some exercise and all would be well in the world. Oh, if it were only that easy. While there is some truth to the fact that a lot of people could easily lose weight if they ate less and got a decent level of exercise, but for many this is just not true. The eat less; get more exercise regime will generally work better for men than women. Can I be bold enough to say that if you are a woman reading this book and you are overweight it is most likely that you are not eating as much food as you should. With the law of averages I see, you will be a small eater. Your ability to train yourself to eat smaller meals is stronger than a typical man. It is very normal for me to find women who are over weight and yet eat very small meals and many times missing meals all because of the belief that if I am too big I must be eating too much. Now I am not suggesting that these same people just need to eat more and they will loose weight. It is not that simple either.

The most important thing about excess weight is to try and

work out why I have this extra weight. Once we know why then it should be easier to correct the problem. So then, is it just the type of food we are eating? No, I don't think it is that simple either because if it were, then why can two people eat the same food and one is overweight and the other one is not. Most people would answer this with the fact that one has a faster metabolism than the other. Just what does that mean; that someone has a fast or slow metabolism. Even if someone does have a slow metabolism why should that make their body turn food into fat? If a person is over eating and consuming twice as many calories as is needed, why should those calories turn into fat? Why don't they just stay in the digestive system and get passed through as waste food or food not needed? Some of these questions have clearly not been answered yet.

Let me repeat my statement that 'I see many people, mainly women, who are very obese, 100kg – 150kg, who are very small eaters'. Some would eat no more than what an average 6 year old child would eat. And they still cannot lose weight. This is because they do not know why they have this excess weight. A reasonable number of people who are overweight will have an excess fluid problem. I covered this in the kidney chapter. It is more common for women to retain excess fluid and it is common for them to have between 4–10 litres of this excess fluid. One litre equals one kilogram, (2.2lbs), and we all know what one litre of water looks like. So it is easy to see what 5 litres of excess fluid would look like in the average body. It takes up a lot of space. If you have a situation where your weight can fluctuate very quickly from day to day then it is most likely that you have an excess fluid problem. Fat cannot come and go from your body on a daily basis at a high level. Get your kidney, renal gland areas working efficiently and this should control the excess fluid.

The main reason I see for a body to be carrying excess fat is the fact that the cells of that body are hungry. If there is a low nutrient level at the cellular level in the body it is very normal for the body to convert food into fat. I have covered this in depth in the chapter on food and digestion. If the food cannot get to the cells to feed them properly, the body knows it will not be able to function to its full capacity for its full life expectancy. The body does not have the ability to get the food to the cells so it will therefore convert that food into fat and store it on the body for possible use later in life. It is somewhat similar to the hibernation process some animals go through. Your body knows that there is a hard time coming later in life, due to the fact that there is insufficient nutrition in the cells, so it feels it needs to store some food away in the form of fat. Weight for weight, fat is a very good energy source your body knows it can fall back on in an emergency.

With most of the health conditions our body can get there are always many different contributing factors as to why you have such a problem, and excess weight is no exception. However, from my experience the single most common reason is a nutrient deficiency at the cellular level. This will not be the low level of just one or two nutrients but a low level of all nutrients. The main reason for having a low nutrient level is our inability to get nutrients from our food because of a very poor digestive system. Once our digestion is up and functioning at a good level it is much easier to get all the required nutrients to our cells. This is when the quality of the food becomes very important. For weight control problems we need to be eating regular meals of low glycaemic foods that are still alive. I have covered this well in the food chapter so please review that information so as to fully understand the very simple things you can do to feed your cells correctly.

There are many weight loss programmes on the market. There are also many wellness programmes. Some of the old weight loss programmes are now called wellness/health programmes. There has been a clear shift away from calling something a weight loss programme to calling it something like wellness or lifestyle. Let's make one point very clear. Just because you lose weight does not mean you are healthier. It is reasonable to presume that if someone is overweight or obese, they could be and probably are unhealthy. They will not necessarily become healthier just because they have lost weight. Many weight control programmes are just short term solutions for long term problems. Some programmes are excellent at helping someone lose weight, but that programme maybe doing more harm than good to the health functions in the body. What I am really trying to say here is please do not judge the health of someone by their weight. When you stand on your scales to weigh yourself understand that those scales can only tell you how heavy an object is. The scales cannot tell you what the object is, whether that object is dead or alive, healthy or not, and whether they are feeling good or not.

For many of us, especially women, the main health measure we use is our weight and shape, or how do I fit my clothes. We believe if only the body size was right I would feel great. For me the three main measures should be:
1.   How do I feel?
2.   How do I function?
3.   How do I fit my clothes? And in that order.

When you get up in the morning ask yourself how do I really feel and at the end of a week, how do I really feel. Be honest with yourself. Then, how does this body function. Does it do what it is supposed to do for its age and stage of life? Are there any aches and pains and is it mechanically fit. Thirdly, can your body fit the clothes size it should? I do know that in most cases if the body is always feeling great because all the functions are going well, then it is relatively easy to get the body to the right size to fit your clothes. Once again we should be looking at getting the whole body healthy rather than just work on one aspect such as the weight of the body.

I have seen many clients lose weight and get back to the desired weight/size using many different programmes. The exciting thing for me when I see them achieving their goal is the fact that they were prepared to give something a good shot. They have been pro-active about a health issue. Remember my first rule about health; 'if there is something not right, do something about it'. I don't care what you do, just do something. So the fact they have done something is great. If you have done something about your weight and have not achieved the required result, don't give up. There will be a solution out there somewhere. Let me repeat what I have seen many times. The main reason for excess weight in a body is poor digestion. Most weight problems are actually well explained in the food chapter. What happens to the food once it gets into your body is more important than what food is going in. Too much time, money and effort is wasted on the very exacting food choices we all should be having rather than what has happened to it once it has been swallowed. So get serious about improving the digestive area of your body. Then also see if your weight problem might resonate with the kidney issues I have shared. Remember that there are many programme/equipment sellers that can quote great weight loss figures, but losing kilograms is not the most important thing and does not paint the full picture of health.

When it comes to which programme I would choose, the only one I now fully endorse is the 'Reset Program'. It is a very complete health programme which should result in a healthy vibrant body. Optimum health is not something one can get from a can or pill, and it is not an instantaneous thing achieved in a few short weeks. Optimum health is a complete lifestyle choice that requires everyday decisions to do the right things to keep well. It does take real commitment to make the correct daily decisions, week in week out for up to 13 months before they will become automatic lifestyle actions that we don't need to think about. We will just do the right thing without thinking about it. An important part of this action is to have fun. Don't be a slave to yourself and take it all too seriously that you miss out on fun. A really good lifestyle programme should be no more than 6 ½ days a week. Some of the most enjoyable things in life don't always come under the good healthy label. Remember that fun itself is a healthy thing.

VIRUSES & BACTERIA

We are currently facing big problems with viruses. Everyday I see and hear of people suffering viral infections at an ever increasing rate. In the work I do on a daily basis I am clearly seeing two distinctive types of virus.

1. The common flu type virus. There are many of these and they are growing in number. More and more people are being affected by common virus all year round, not just winter time. When there is a common virus in the body, the body will nearly always recognise it as a virus and there will be an immune system response to that virus, either a temperature change or mucus production in the breathing passages.

2. There is a large growth in the occurrence of a different type of virus. The main thing that makes this virus different from a common flu virus is the fact that your immune system cannot identify that it is a virus, so there will be very little effort by the body to eliminate it, or should I say a confused effort. The body will nearly always know that there is something wrong but it will not know what it is, therefore it won't know which immune system response to activate.

For this reason a virus of this type can then stay in the body for a long time and do a lot of damage, for weeks, months and even years. I measure virus on a frequency scale and the higher the frequency, the less likely it is that your body will identify the virus.

Generally speaking a virus is a very small organism only about 1/300 the size of a bacteria. This gives the virus the ability to penetrate through the membranes of a cell into the nucleus area of that cell. A virus is not a complete cell on its own so it needs another cell to live in. A virus will mainly live in the nucleus of a cell, whereas a bacteria is a complete cell so all it needs is food and a nice environment to live in and it can then multiply and spread throughout the body. This is when our immune system will identify it as a foreign body and try to eliminate it.

Most viruses are very particular as to what cell they would like to live in. Some can only survive in a heart cell, or liver cell, or lung cell etc.

The main way our body will eliminate a virus is with temperature. Most viruses can only live in a 2 C degree range of temperature, so if your body has identified that there is a virus in the body and it is at a bad level the body temperature will increase by 3-4 C degree so as to kill the virus. That is why when we have the flu we get a temperature, sometimes we even feel very cold but our temperature is up. If your body can hold the temperature 3-4 C degree above normal for a day or two the virus will be killed. So if you have the flu, go to bed and sweat it out.

One way to kill a common virus quickly is by having an herbal tea made with ginger and sage. Use the root ginger. Cut a slice off the root ginger and place it in a cup. Then add a leaf or two of fresh sage or ½ a teaspoon of dried sage. Boil the kettle and then pour the water into the cup. It's as simple as that. Have up to a maximum of 6 cups, maybe three cups one day then three cups the next. This simple tea will eliminate most common virus. To further enhance this tea you could do the following. In a saucepan put 4-5 cups of water and then add 3-4 slices root ginger, 3-4 leaves of sage, 1 teaspoon of honey and one whole lemon. Cut the lemon and squeeze it into the water, then put the whole lemon in with the other ingredients and bring them up to boiling point. Simmer for 15–20 minutes then drink. This should have a very immediate impact to clear the virus.

There are many other benefits to this brew. The ginger is very good for the liver which in turn plays a big part in supporting our immune system. It can sometimes help settle digestion problems. Ginger tea is also very good for emotional issues. The sage is very good at boosting ones metabolism and can also benefit the hormonal function. This herbal tea should never be microwaved. It will never work if it has been microwaved. The life force of food is always destroyed when anything is microwaved. Just boil the kettle and pour the water on. You can drink this tea hot, warm or cold. Do not have more than 5-6 cups of sage tea at any given time. It should just be a short sharp dose every now and then. A fresh brew should be made each day.

A virus will do a lot of damage to the inside of a cell. This can only be repaired when we are sleeping. Nearly all the repair in our body gets done when we are sleeping, so if there has been a lot of damage done in a body, e.g. viral damage, we will need to get more sleep than normal so as to repair those damaged cells. Thus the body will send you the tired signal so you might go to sleep so some repair might take place. The greater the damage, the greater the tired signal.

How many times do we see a person that is tired and generally unwell, go for a check-up at the doctor, just to get told that it is probably a virus? Go home and rest. The doctor is many times right, but can't always prove this. It is very common to have an underlying virus in the body that cannot be measured by a doctor.

Now, let us take this a step further and look at the growing number of the unusual types of virus I mentioned earlier. Your body is being damaged at the cellular level so it will be trying to repair, thus it will be more tired than usual. These unusual viruses are doing a lot of damage but the immune system does not know it is a virus so there will be no specific immune system response to this negative activity. The virus keeps doing its damage. The body keeps trying to repair the damage by asking for more sleep. Because the body cannot identify it as a virus, the virus will continue to live freely in the body for a long time. The most common case of this is Chronic Fatigue or Tapanui Flu, but there are many other examples.

I do not know of any simple way of eliminating these type of virus accept with a high frequency vibration. This is a specialized field. There are many different machines in use that may help with this type of viral problem. The best I have seen is when the virus can be clearly identified, so then it can be treated with the exact right frequency. There are many different ways of doing this, but it would be best to leave this to explain in more detail later. There are many cases where just the time factor does finally allow the immune system to do its job and kill the virus, sometimes by pure luck. High doses of some nutrients such as vitamins C, and E or garlic, and some other herbal plants can work well at times.

There is one herbal tea which has shown a high level of success with these viruses. It is mullein tea. Any good herbalist shop should stock mullein in a dried leaf form. Check it out and use as recommended. It just might do the trick in cases where there is continued tiredness for which there is no explanation.

The best way to avoid bacterial and viral infections is to have a good healthy life style. My basic rules of life are the first thing to look at. These are explained in detail in the final chapter. Good food, good digestion, good liver and kidneys and a healthy exercise programme.

Bacteria are easier to avoid than virus. The single biggest factor I see with the viral problems is a person's genetic make-up. The quality of our genes really is an open lottery. Genetic selection is out of our control. The quality of our genetic make-up has the greatest determining factor over whether we will be likely to get viral infections or not. We can't control this genetic make up, but regardless of our genetic quality we still have the choice of how well we look after our cells.

Bacteria

Most of the time, if your body has a bacterial infection at a bad level, it will nearly always be able to identify this so there will be an immune system response to this. Thus you will know something is wrong. Generally the best medicine for bacterial infections is an antibiotic. If used properly and wisely antibiotic are fantastic, but if over-used they can be very damaging. Antibiotic are the best solution for a lot of bacteria but are usually of very little help with viral problems.

One very simple solution for a few bacterial infections is chives tea. For any bacterial infections in the digestion system, kidneys, bladder, urinary tract, or blood system, chives tea usually works a treat. Just put 2-3 stalks of chive into a cup and poor on the hot water from your kettle. Do not microwave this tea. Maximum dose is 4 cups, and try to consume this within two days. Chives are in the same family as garlic and we have known for centuries the value of garlic.

Check out the chapter on Solutions. There are many different things you can try for the elimination of an infection which are very simple, and when you get the right one, very effective.

From my measuring and experiences, I see garlic as a great immune system support and very good to prevent an infection entering the body, especially bacteria. However, garlic is not so good at killing an infection once you have it at a bad level. Chives are a great killer of bugs but of little value in protection like the garlic. Garlic strengthens and supports the immune system.

When the bacterial infection is in a more specific area like the throat or ears, eyes or nose, the chives is not so good. There are many herbal and natural medicines that can work well in this area but if you are not getting the result you need quickly, check it out at your GP and look at the antibiotic solution. Be sensible. You all know the rule – if symptoms persist, seek medical advice.

MICROWAVE COOKING & ELECTROMAGNETIC FIELDS

There is a lot of confusing information out there about the safety of microwaving your food. What I will share with you is my personal opinion based on what I have read and seen. Using a microwave and being exposed to electromagnetic radiation can be damaging to our health and usually is. I am not a fan of microwaves and recommend that we do not use a microwave on a regular base. It is a very similar situation to the smoking issue. Some people can smoke until they are 90 years old and have no apparent negative effect from that smoking. Others who smoke can end up with lung or throat cancer at 35 years of age. It is not worth the risk of smoking and I feel the same about using a microwave to cook your food.

The way a microwave works is like this. There is a particular electromagnetic frequency produced by the machine that is very reactive on water molecules. This frequency is radiated into the microwave box. It then makes the positive and negative electrons around the nucleus of water molecules in the food rotate. These electrons rotate very fast which will then create a fast changing polarity in the nucleus of each cell. This changing polarity makes the nucleus explode creating heat. Water molecules are the most receptive to this type of radiation. When there are a lot of the cells in the food exploding in the nucleus, there is collectively enough heat to make the whole dish of food hot. This in turn destroys all the life in the cell. The main life force of the cell has just been destroyed. Laboratory tests may show good levels of vitamins and minerals but they cannot test to see how much life is left in the food. Foods that have been microwaved will have very little life left in them, whether they have been cooked properly or just re-heated. Cooking and re-heating are exactly the same process, cooking just takes a little longer. This electron reaction will continue happening in the food for up to three minutes after the machine has stopped. This is why it is recommended to stand the food for a few minutes until the reaction stops.

Normal heat is created through friction. As one cell gets hot it vibrates faster and faster. This is rubbed off onto the next cell and on it goes. It is just friction at a high level and mostly this will not destroy the life force of the cell. This is a slower form of heating something, but safer. The microwave is just more convenient. The word convenient is just a long way of spelling lazy. We do things the convenient way because we are too lazy to do it the proper way.

The worst use of a microwave that I have seen is the heating of a baby's milk bottle. It will destroy the life of the food with the result being that the infant will be under-nourished. Please realise that for a young one on a bottle, all of its food will be coming via the microwave as verses for an adult, microwaved food will probably be only a small portion of the total diet. In such cases the infant is usually rather unhappy and needing to be fed often.

Because the radiation is still in the milk, the stomach will be getting damaged. There are very small amounts of radiation left in that food, and this radiation can be very harsh on the digestive enzymes and bacteria in the stomach. This will cause discomfort that will most times appear like serious wind or colic. Many times the easiest way to settle the baby is to give it more of the same food. The baby will always show signs of hunger because at the cellular level it is hungry due to the poor quality food and the poor digestion. The infant will many times have a large stomach and be putting on weight so mother will presume her child is well fed. Because the young one is under nourished it will not be able to sleep for long periods, so will wake more often. It will be looking for and needing more food. It is another one of these vicious cycles, where the quality of the food is creating the problem, and then the under-nourished body wanting more of that food. Stop the microwaved bottle, warm it in hot water, and see a new infant within ten days. It will be sleeping longer, be more peaceful and needing less food.

Any food or drink that we consume from a microwave that is still hot will have some residual microwave radiation in it. This radiation may have a detrimental effect on the enzymes and bacteria in our stomach that digest our food. This in turn may have a very negative effect on our ability to get nutrients from our food to nourish our cells.

The main issue here is when we consume something on a very regular basis from our microwave, i.e. porridge for breakfast everyday; babies bottle every meal; that coffee warmed up at the office 5-6 times a day. There is a two fold effect here. One is the lower quality food and the other is the possible damage to your digestive system. Porridge has a good ability to hold this microwave radiation and when you eat your porridge each morning it is the first thing your stomach has received since last night. Those enzymes in your stomach that digest your food have had nothing to eat since last night's dinner so they are hungry. The first food they receive each day, everyday, contains microwave radiation. This is not good.

Another issue with the microwave is when we heat up the wheat bag for pain relief. When it is hot and we place it on our body it is still radiating out microwave radiation. The heat might feel nice and soothing but the radiation can negate any of those benefits, especially around the head and brain area. It is my strongest recommendation not to use the wheat bag in this area on a regular basis. A hot water bottle is much safer. There is also the option of some of the more specialised heat packs you can get that don't need to be microwaved. Some chemists and physiotherapists supply these.

A handy tip I once heard on the TV was how to get rid of all those bugs in your kitchen bench cloth. Wet the cloth and then put it in the microwave on high for one minute, it will kill all the bugs. If it can do that in one minute to the dish cloth, what will it do to your food if it is in there for 5 minutes or longer? How can anything in your food still be alive?

The topic of electromagnetic radiation and the associated negative side effects has been well published in books and documentaries that most of us have seen or heard. If you have regular exposure to electromagnetic radiation I am very sure in the belief that it will have a negative effect on your health. I have seen it so many times in every day situations having a very clear negative effect on a person's immune system and brain function. To find out more of the details about how this can affect your health you need to get down to the library or search the internet. There is a wealth of information to be found but many times it can get very complicated for the average person without a scientific background. Let me briefly explain how it works.

Our bodies are electric. It is electric currents feeding from the brain that make our body function. There are millions of electric signals sent around the body at all times of the day and night keeping all parts of the body functioning in the right way. If the body is exposed to high levels of man-made electric fields it is very likely that these fields will interfere with our body's own electric system. It really is as simple as that. There is no need for me to go into all the detail of how this happens. It is just very important to know that damage to your cells can and probably will happen if you spend too much time being exposed to electromagnetic radiation.

Most of us are well aware of the negativity from large power pylons and therefore would choose not to live near them. Well there are many cases where the radiation in the typical bedroom can be just as bad as living under a pylon and therefore very damaging on a persons health.

There is only one main rule to remember when you have concerns about electromagnetic radiation. It is all about time and distance. How close are you to the field and for how long? The strength of the radiation is not as significant as how close are you to it and how much time are you spending in that radiation zone.

In many bedrooms there are electrical appliances all around the bed; electric blanket, clock radio, lamps, water beds with electric heaters, TV, computer, stereo sound systems, and many other gadgets that we think are essential for good living. Then out of sight you may be exposed to the radiation from an appliance through the wall at the head of the bed such as refrigerator, freezer, TV, power switch board, electric wire circuits in the wall, TV satellite dish, power inlet to the house, and street power transformers in close proximity to the house. The list is long and varied.

Most of these potential hazards have a lower radiation than a large power pylon, but the problem is the amount of time you spend in close proximity to these appliances while in your bed, and how close you are to the radiation source. We spend around

8 hours or 1/3 of our lives in the one place called a bed. There is no other location in our daily lives where we will spend that much time in one exact spot. Some of this electrical equipment can be very close to the body or even right against the body for that full 8 hours.

The electric blanket and clock radio are potentially the worst because of the distance factor. The electric blanket is hard against the whole body all night. The electric blanket should always be un-plugged while we sleep. The clock radio is usually very close to the head.

Now think of the distance factor. All other appliances should be at least 6 feet from our bodies, especially the head/brain area. In the chapter on sleep you will see just what happens at sleep time and how it is the brain that does all the important things at this time. Over head power-lines and transformers within 20-30 metres of a bedroom can be very bad for anyone but especially young children.

In the work place there can be many electrical appliances and machines that are impossible to avoid. If this is the case the most important thing to do is regularly earth yourself out. Every 20-30 minutes you need to go and touch some metal object like a water tap or the bare earth. This can allow your body to discharge any electricity that has been building up in your body. This earthing will have a very positive affect on your immune system. When you leave work each day try to find a place where you can be in contact with the earth. When you get home walk bare foot on the ground.

In most office buildings the atmosphere is very positively charged because of all of the electrical equipment. This positively charged air is not good for our immune system. We need air with a negative ion charge. The best negative air we can get is from beside the sea. As the air moves over the ocean it is negatively charged which will boost our immune system. How many times at the end of a day do we feel low on energy but when we go for a good walk along the beach we can come back energized. Negative ions charge us up while positive ions take away our energy.

When it comes to electromagnetic fields the best thing we can do is practise prudent avoidance. Make your sleep area clear of all electrical junk. Be aware of any high voltage electricity around your house and work place. Keeping physically fit will help protect you from some of the dangers.

The most common symptom to suffer when you are exposed to bad electric fields is tiredness, headaches and general brain tension. These are very general symptoms that many people will experience for lots of different reasons.

Because a child's body is growing while it sleeps it is very important that we have a clean and safe area for them to sleep in. There are many studies that indicate there could be a close connection between electromagnetic fields and childhood leukaemia. Prudent avoidance is very cheap.

Cell phones and cell phone towers can be harmful. We really don't know so much about these issues but recent studies have shown that we should be concerned, especially for the long term prospects of ill health. I personally have seen young people with decreasing health once they became exposed to cell phone tower radiations. Sometimes the effect has been very harsh and very quick. Cell phones should not be kept in our bed with us while we sleep. The radiation from a cell phone that is turned on and kept close to the brain will penetrate well into the brain.

The younger the person is the further the radiation will penetrate through the brain. The biggest issue here is the fact that we just do not know what possible long term negative affects there may be on our health with this technology. Too many young ones are using their cell phone to text their friends all night so therefore keep the cell phone under their pillow. This could be a very dangerous practice.

There are many things in relation to electromagnetic radiation that I would like to cover here but there is no point. It would take a full book. I have covered the most important things and I would very much encourage you just to be aware of the dangers and try to avoid long term exposure of any electromagnetic radiations.

Don't presume that these radiations are safe just because you cannot feel them. There is enough anecdotal and scientific evidence showing the potential danger to our health. Understanding the sleep process is very important when considering these electromagnetic fields. The two are closely connected. Lets now look at what sleep is all about and how it works.

CHAPTER NINE
SLEEP

If the sun wouldn't go behind
The curtains at night,
How would earth be illuminated
in the Morning?
Rumi

Sleep is one of the most important functions of a human body. It is the time when we repair our cells. Nearly all of our cell repair and replication for growth takes place while we sleep. When we are awake the cell replication process is getting ready for full on action when we fall asleep. The cell repair process is similar to cell replication for growth from the point of view that the cell is dividing into two and then growing to full size so as to do its function in your body.

There are millions of cells that have to be repaired or replaced in your body each day. All of this replication is controlled by the brain. It is beyond comprehension just how complicated this process must be. Millions and millions of cells are replaced every day and all controlled by the brain. This is the most important job your brain does because without it we would degenerate very fast. Nearly all of this regeneration takes place when we sleep so getting quality sleep is essential for good health. We need to get enough time sleeping and that sleep should be good quality sleep.

The main regeneration takes place when we get into our delta sleep. If things are working well we should get approximately 6-8 delta periods in our sleep each night. The delta is a very deep sleep of about 10-15 minutes. This is when there is a large amount of activity happening in the body as cells are replicating. In between each delta sleep is the rem (rapid eye movement) sleep.

Of all the work your brain does nearly 70% will be while we sleep. All of our awake time only contributes to about 30% of the work your brain does. Most of you might be surprised to hear this but it just shows how much activity happens in your body while you sleep.

Let's expand that further. We spend 1/3 of our time sleeping and 2/3 of our time awake. The 1/3 of our time sleeping is when the brain does 70% of its work and it has 2/3 of the time to do only 30% of its work. If you think the brain is busy during the day, just look how busy it is at sleep time. At sleep time it has only half the time to do more than double the work that it does during wake time. This equates to the brain working at least 4 times faster when we are sleeping.

When we go to sleep our brain wakes up to do its main work. If the brain cannot wake up properly to do this work our body won't be able to get into the sleep mode. Many people have trouble getting to sleep and comment that their brain is too active and will not slow down so they can't get to sleep. Actually, it is just the opposite of that. Because the brain cannot wake up and get into full function our body cannot fall asleep.

There are many different reasons why the brain cannot get

active enough so as to put you into the sleep mode. The most common reasons I see are:

1. Bad location of bed
2. Insufficient nutrient in the brain cells
3. Bad pH level in the brain cells
4. Mental stress

The location of your bed is very important. For many years we have known of a thing called geopathic stress that can interfere with our sleep. Geo- meaning something from the earth and -pathic meaning pathogen, something bad. So geopathic stress is something coming from the ground that is bad for us if we are exposed to it for too long. For many of us we will view this topic with a high level of suspicion and I do respect everyone's freedom to choose what they want to believe in or not. However, from my 25 years experience in this field I have no doubt of the reality of geopathic stress.

The most common form of geopathic stress is under ground water streams. This is easily checked by an experienced diviner/ dowser. How can under ground water effect us, you may ask? Any water that is continually flowing in the same direction will draw gravity to it. There will be an increased level of gravitational pull above any water that is continually flowing in the same direction.

Gravity is a magnetic field that is pulling everything to the earth. It is just one big magnet in the core of the earth that pulls everything towards the earths centre. If we are exposed to a higher level of gravity, magnetic pull, than what is standard, for prolonged periods it can interfere with our immune system. The most common place that we can get long term exposure to this form of geopathic stress is in our bed. We spend about 1/3 of our life in bed, on the same spot. Other than the bed it is unlikely anyone will spend that amount of time in any other location.

When we are sleeping we are trying to repair our cells from the day's activity and general wear and tear. This is controlled by the brain sending millions of electrical signals around the body telling the right cells to replicate in the right quantity. The brain knows which cells and how many cells need attention.

The sleep process is all electrical, so if the body is exposed to an electric or magnetic field when it is trying to sleep it may make the sleep process difficult. The brain will then have to spend too much of the sleep time trying to protect you from this radiation rather than repairing you. Most of the time the geopathic stress we experience will be a magnetic field, but not always.

There are many different types of geopathic stress, too many to talk about here. But rest assured geopathic stress is real and it can have a very negative effect on most people who have long term exposure to it. Geopathic stress is a complete book on its own, with many variations of type and strength, too much to talk about here.

Something very similar to geopathic in the sleep area is electromagnetic stress. It has a similar negative effect on a sleeping body but will come from man-made electricity. Common issues are clock radios, electric blankets, water bed heaters, electrical appliances close to the bed, power pylons and transformers close to the house, meter boards close to the bed and some television aerials. Any of these have potential to interfere with our sleep process, because of the electromagnetic fields they radiate, so prudent avoidance is best option. Once again for me, this is another book just to cover all the possibilities in this area.

Most of the time exposure to geopathic and electromagnetic stress will make it hard to get to sleep. So if you find you are tired enough to sleep but just can't get to sleep it maybe because of the location of your bed. Common sense says shift the bed to another position or try sleeping in another bed to see what happens. Even try putting the pillow at the foot end of the bed. Sometimes there may be a water stream running under the head of the bed so put your head at the other end and see what happens. It will cost you nothing to try it.

Bed wetting is a very common symptom when children sleep above water streams. Try moving the bed or moving to another position. If you find your child moves to the opposite end of a bed or curls up in one spot all the time, it will probably be because your child is moving away from a bad spot. So when you see your child at the wrong end of the bed don't pull them back to the correct position. Leave them where they are. They have probably found the best spot.

The depth of an underground water stream does not affect its strength. Its strength is determined by how much water is flowing past that spot. The greater the volume, the greater the negative effect will be.

For a healing body or a growing body the quality of the location is very important. There is growing evidence of the connection between some childhood cancers and electromagnetic fields. Other studies have shown a strong correlation between under ground water streams and cancer. To find out more check it out at your local library or look on the internet. The evidence is rather compelling. But the big issue here is that it is so easy to avoid the problem. If in doubt shift the sleep position and see what happens.

Sleep is a function. While part of the reason for sleeping is to give the body a rest, the main point is regeneration of cells. This is a process that takes time and for most of us that sleep process speed is very similar so we will need a good 8 hours sleep if we want to get all that function done properly each night.

There are a very small number of people who can sleep faster than normal so will need less time in the sleep mode. Similarly there are some who sleep slow so will need a good 10 hours each night. Children need more sleep than an adult because they have normal repair to do like us but they also need to make many new cells for growth. It is the same after a big surgery or illness. We need to make many new cells and can only do this when we sleep so we need to get that extra sleep.

If the nutrient level in the body is low it will be hard for a person to stay asleep for the full time needed. We do consume a large amount of energy while we sleep. When we start our sleep with a low level of energy in the body we will run out of that energy before all the sleep process has been done. There is a difference between being tired and being low on energy. Most of us have never thought of this so will not appreciate the difference.

So it is important to have a descent quantity of good food later in the day. Belief has it that we should have our main meal of the day as the mid-day meal and then have a lighter meal at the end of the day. This is mainly because of our inability to digest the food properly and we are more likely to turn that food into fat if we go to bed on a full stomach. I do not agree with this. I have covered the fat issue in the chapter on weight control. We do need a good level of food later in the day so as to have the required nutrients for good sleep.

Our body has the ability to use our food very quickly after we have eaten. How many times have we felt very tired within 30 minutes of having our mid-day meal? This is the body responding to the nutrient arriving in the blood. The brain then says it wants to use this food for repair rather than you using the food for body movement. We can only repair when we are asleep, so now that there is some good nutrient just arrived, the brain will say please go to sleep so the nutrient can be used for some repair. Does this make sense and sound logical.

When we have our power naps after lunch for 20-30 minutes we can get a huge amount of cell replication done in a very short time period. Power naps can be very useful and have a positive outcome whereas a nana nap is slower and somewhat negative. It says I am getting old and need a rest, whereas the power nap says I just need a quick sleep so as to get going at full speed again. Be well aware of the power of the mind.

It is very common to have a low nutrient level in our cells and most of this was covered in the chapters on food, digestion, liver and kidneys. Of all the different nutrients we require for optimum health calcium is the most important for sleep. Nearly all of the calcium we consume will be metabolised at sleep time. If we are low on calcium it will be hard to stay asleep for the full duration needed.

Typically as we age our calcium levels get very low and our calcium storage in the bones become a serious problem. We see this clearly with the osteoporosis statistics. Many people as they age think they don't need as much sleep. This is very much supported by the fact that most of the elderly can't sleep as long as they used to, although they are still very tired. The main reason they cannot sleep right through the night is the fact that there is just not enough calcium in the body to allow good sleep.

If you have a sleep pattern where you are tired enough to go to sleep and have no trouble getting to sleep but find that you regularly wake at the same time in the early hours of the morning it will nearly always be because of a lack of calcium available for proper sleep process. So the obvious solution is to take a good calcium supplement. Magnesium is an essential nutrient to have with calcium so make sure your supplement has both of these nutrients. It is always best to take this supplement at night time. The magnesium is good for relaxing the body.

There is however one major issue here. If you think you are low in calcium or have had tests to check bone density and have clinical proof of low levels, it makes sense to take a supplement to make up for the down fall.

Why is it then, that we hardly ever ask the question of 'why am I low in calcium in the first place'. Low calcium levels will nearly always be because of poor digestion, inefficient kidneys or low liver function. Most of us do have enough calcium going onto our bodies but lack the ability to extract and absorb it. This is true for all the other nutrients we require for optimum cellular function.

If you get your digestion and kidneys working better with the solutions I recommend you will get a much better sleep; longer, deeper and more settled. Which means you will wake more refreshed and able to face a new day with great energy and enthusiasm.

If your kidney or liver function is poor it will interfere with the sleep process, particularly the liver. It creates a high acid level in the blood which in turn has a very negative effect on brain function. Poor kidneys will make you very tired, and then it does not matter how much sleep you get, you will still be tired. It becomes a vicious cycle.

Mental stress and worries can be very bad for sleep but are seldom permanent or long term. There are many things in the herbal and nutritional line that can help with mental stress as well as good food and exercise. I must stress here though that the most common reason for long term sleep problems will be either a location problem or a lack of nutrient in the body at the cellular level.

Sleep is all about repair and regeneration of your cells, so if you are not getting enough sleep or the quality of your sleep is poor you will be degenerating faster than you should. An accelerated aging will most likely bring in a degenerative disease for you.

Most of us will spend too many years of our life suffering from a degenerative disease; i.e. cancer, heart disease, Alzheimer's, arthritis, osteoporosis, diabetes, MS, etc, etc. So make the effort to be sure the quality of your sleep is perfect. Be pro-active in your efforts to achieve this perfect regeneration time. Life is too short not to.
Sleep tight.

HEART DISEASE

Heart disease is the scourge of the western world. It is affecting nearly every family in a very direct way. We all have family members or friends who have had a heart attack, have blood pressure problems or out of control cholesterol. Many of our elderly friends are suffering circulation problems. Much research has been done and millions of dollars have been spent to find the reason and the solution and yet these problems still run rampant. Most of the medical efforts revolve around control of the situation rather than the cause. Let me give a very down to earth view of the cause of heart disease. This will then connect with a solution for those who are living with heart disease, high cholesterol or circulation problems.

The most common reason people suffer any form of heart disease is because the circulation of the blood around our body is very poor. Let me at this stage point out a very important issue. There is a big difference between circulation of the blood verses blood quality. Circulation is a measure of how freely your blood flows through your blood vessels. Many times someone will have poor blood and feel it as poor circulation, when in fact the blood might be circulating perfect. This was high-lighted in the chapter on kidney function. Some of the most common reasons for poor quality blood are; poor kidney function, poor liver function, a virus or bacteria in the blood system, chemicals in the blood, and poor spleen function.

When we have poor circulation one common symptom is cold hands and feet and slight discolouration of the skin. This is because there is a poor supply of blood to the skin. Enough blood just can't get there. The same symptoms will be experienced if the quality of the blood is bad. The blood can get to the skin but it has poor nutrients and a low level of oxygen, so in reality it is the same situation as far as the cell is concerned. In both scenarios the body cell is lacking in vital nutrients and low levels of oxygen, but for two completely different reasons, which require two completely different solutions.

Therefore given a situation where someone has a bad case of common heart disease, there can be more than one reason for having that problem; poor blood or bad circulation or both. The most common reason I see for having poor quality blood is having poor kidney function. I covered this well in the kidney chapter and offered some solutions there. A low spleen will have a big influence over the blood quality. There is a close relationship between the liver and the spleen, so if the spleen is down in function it may be because of the liver. Check out the section on the liver for guidance. There can be many other reasons the quality of the blood is poor but for the purpose of this book I want to share with you the main common reasons people have these problems.

Circulation, the ability of the blood to flow through our arteries and veins, is a very large and concerning problem. Typically as we age our circulation gets worse and there is even an expectation that it has to deteriorate. This does not have to be the case. The most common reason for blood flow restriction is fatty deposits blocking the blood vessel and or hardening of the blood vessel wall. We get told that 'fatty foods block the blood vessels, so keep off fatty foods'. Not true. What is clearly understood now is the fact that oxidation of the cholesterol is the main reason we build up this fatty plaque in our blood vessels.

Cholesterol levels in the blood stream have been used as a measure for heart disease. High cholesterol has been an indicator of a bad situation. Then it was said that the main problem was if your bad cholesterol – LDL- was too high. This cholesterol is very easily oxidized which will cause it to coagulate and cling to the blood vessel wall creating a restriction to the blood flow.

Free radical oxygen molecules in the blood are responsible for most of our oxidative damage, hence the need for a high level of antioxidants in our diet. These antioxidants should mainly come from fresh alive food, but it is well advised to consider taking a high quality antioxidant supplement as well. Research is now saying that the main culprit is VLDL. This is a very small, dense LDL particle which is showing to be very good at hardening the blood vessel walls. To find out more detail on this topic check out www.releasingfat.com. It has a wealth of information on heart disease and related issues.

Despite all of this science, I do believe there are more important issues that need looking at. There does seem to be a very clear push from medical authorities to lower the level of cholesterol. They say that if we get the cholesterol level down we will fix a lot of this heart disease problem. They seem more concerned with getting the level down rather than finding out why it is high in the first place.

Most people will scream out loudly that the cholesterol level is high because of what we eat and a lack of good exercise. Too many fatty foods and highly processed foods combined with a sedentary life style. Sure, there are people who do improve their lifestyle choices that have their cholesterol level drop but, there are just as many who make very good lifestyle decisions and yet don't have their level drop.

Too many people take medications to lower their cholesterol level and it works well, but they still do not know why their cholesterol was high in the first place. Both doctor and patient are happy because the cholesterol is at the safer level so all must be well. If the reason for having the high cholesterol is still there then we can presume that a problem still exists. High cholesterol is the body's way of saying there is something wrong. It is like a red light on the dash board. The prescribed medication is usually just a good way to turn off the warning light by cutting the wire that leads to it, rather than getting to the source of the problem.

Medical studies have started to understand what cholesterol does in our body but they do not know why some of us produce higher levels of cholesterol compared to others. What is very important to me is not so much the level of cholesterol in our body but why is it there and even more importantly what is happening to the cholesterol I do have. Is it being oxidized by free radicals or not?

Having a high level of cholesterol that is not being oxidized is of little concern compared with of very low level of cholesterol with a high oxidation rate. So first and foremost keep up a high level of antioxidants so as to control the oxidation damage. But still we need to look back further and find out why so many of us are producing very high levels of cholesterol.

Let me give you my theory. For me cholesterol is the opposite of adrenalin. Adrenalin is a hormone we produce in the adrenal glands to deal with stress and fright and flight. When we need to physically act at a quick level of response we will produce more adrenalin so as to speed the body up. We can produce this adrenalin at will, very quickly.

Cholesterol is the opposite. When we need to get calmed down we will produce extra cholesterol. We can produce cholesterol very instantly, so we need to see cholesterol as a tranquilizer, something to calm us down. If our cholesterol level is high it will nearly always be because our body is stressed about something. Stressed is a very broadly used word here. If anything is functioning poorly in your body that your body is concerned about then your body will most likely produce more cholesterol. Take as an example the situation of someone having a heart attack, surviving the attack, being taken to a hospital and having the usual tests. One of the first things the emergency people do is to place a drip supply into the blood stream with magnesium. Magnesium's most immediate function is to calm the body down. It is a tranquilizer.

The first blood test will usually show high levels of cholesterol so therefore it is presumed the high cholesterol was the cause of the heart attack. The medical people have seen this scenario many thousand times over many years, so it would be logical to presume that cholesterol caused the problem.

Having cholesterol oxidized will help to create the heart disease but in many cases the very high cholesterol is caused because of the heart attack. That sudden near death experience is a huge stress on the body so it will produce a lot more cholesterol to calm the body down. At any stage of any day if you get a very sudden scare in any way, your body will increase the production of cholesterol instantly. Our bodies are very good at producing cholesterol on demand.

Many people have a high cholesterol level all the time. This will be because there is a permanent stress going on in their body all the time. Poor kidneys and low liver are the two most common reasons I see for long term stress inside the body, but there are many other reasons your body will feel stressed enough to continually produce cholesterol at a high level. Some of these include; bad sleep position, not enough sleep, to much exercise, chemical affects, mental stress, poor nutrient level, emotional problems, long term viral infection, poor circulation, over weight, under weight, electromagnetic radiation, bad prescription drugs, and the list goes on.

For some people the sight of a needle at the doctors for a blood test can cause anxiety which can instantly elevate the cholesterol level and blood pressure reading. This is commonly called white coat syndrome. The frustration of having high cholesterol and trying to get it down without success, then having to go for your regular check up knowing that your doctor is going to tell you again that you need to get it lower, usually with the same information of lifestyle changes and continue with the medication. Many patients are trying very hard, but the doctor makes them feel very inadequate, so they get up-tight when they visit their doctor, which pushes up the cholesterol level, which further justifies the doctor's comments, which then further upsets the patient. It is a vicious circle.

The main medications recommended by medical practitioners are statin drugs. These are very commonly used around the world to control cholesterol levels. From what I understand, one of the main functions of this drug is to calm the body down or what some people feel, slow it down.

How this works is it has the ability to slow down the production and function of Co-enzyme Q10. This is an enzyme that makes our energy work. Crudely speaking, CoQ10 is the flame we put on petrol to create heat. Without the flame the petrol creates no heat/energy. Petrol is a source of energy that has not been activated until a flame is put in it. Without Co-enzyme Q10 there is nothing to turn our energy into heat. Our energy cannot work, so we will feel low in energy and somewhat lethargic.

A lot of people who take statin drugs experience these symptoms of low energy. If the body is working at a slower pace, because of the lowered Co-enzyme Q10, it will usually produce less cholesterol because it feels calmer. So we can see how statin drugs can lower our body's production of cholesterol which will please the doctor. But we still have not got to the cause for having high cholesterol in the first place. And have we dealt with the oxidation of the cholesterol yet? No we have not. It is another situation of the symptom is better so the problem must be gone. In reality it is just a good plaster on a festering wound. We have only covered up the problem.

We need to take a different approach to cholesterol. Don't be so worried about how high your cholesterol is, but rather try and find out why it is so high. Look at the three main problems I see; digestion, liver, and kidneys. If you do have high cholesterol it will be because your body feels it is stressed. There will be a function within the body not working well. High cholesterol will very seldom be because of something outside of the body, and remember cholesterol is not the main problem. Cholesterol is an indication of a problem. Cholesterol is the red warning light trying to indicate to us that something else is going wrong.

If you do have cholesterol problems and/or blood pressure issues there are several things you should immediately do. Firstly start taking a high quality omega 3 oil. There are many of these on the market with the most common being either fish oil or flaxseed oil. There are many different plant seed oils that are good for this solution.

Taking good quantities of a quality oil can significantly reduce the amount of fatty plaque build up in our blood vessels. This is the quickest and most simple way to make more space in our blood vessels for the blood to travel through so as to carry our nutrients around the body to our cells and then get the rubbish and carry it out. When we are taking good omega 3 oils there are two quite different scenarios. The first is taking an oil to try and fix something and the second is taking good oil for maintaining good health. If we are trying to fix a circulation problem we need to be taking 2–3 times more oil than what is needed for maintenance. For the problem solving application I recommend taking oil on a spoon instead of in a capsule so as to get enough volume into the system. For maintenance 1-2 capsules are usually fine.

When there is a circulation problem it is very common to be prescribed medications that thin the blood down so that it can flow through the blood vessels more easily. While this can be life saving in the short term, don't you think it would make sense to try and clean out the blood vessels so more blood can get through. Have a bigger hole for the blood to pass through rather than making the blood thinner to fit through the small hole.

Another issue here is, if the medical tests can see that your main arteries are blocked, what are the smaller capillaries like. The arteries are mainly there for the movement of blood to the smaller vessels where the blood then passes the oxygen and nutrients into the cell. From this point one could say that the smaller capillaries are more important than the bigger arteries and veins. They are all important. But if the bigger vessels are showing signs of blockage you can be sure the smaller ones are suffering even more. So consume lots of oil.

The second solution is getting your digestion working well. Take a look at the chapter on food and digestion. This can play a huge role in reducing the stress levels in any body. Getting a good level of exercise 3-4 times a week helps to pump blood through your arteries and veins at a higher rate than usual. This can help clean out the fatty plaque build-up.

The heart is a pump. Its job is to pump blood around your body through all the blood vessels. If the blood vessels are getting blocked it will be harder for the heart to pump the blood. This will usually result in the heart beating faster than normal. You will have an increased heart rate.

If you can get yourself a healthy exercise programme in place combined with a good diet and supplementation of omega 3 oils you should be able to clean-out some of the fatty deposits in your blood vessels. This should make it easier for the heart to pump the blood. If your heart rate drops from 78 beats per minute to 77 beats per minute you have saved the heart more than 525,600 beats each year. That's more than half a million less beats of the heart each year just by reducing the heart rate by one beat per minute. If you lowered the heart rate by 5 beats per minute that is 2.5 million less beats each year. This has got to have a big positive effect on the heart. The pump should last a lot longer.

In the last chapter I have my basic rules for good health. If you do these well there should be a very significant reduction in heart disease symptoms, blood pressure problems and cholesterol issues.

JOINTS & ARTHRITIS

Traditionally seen as an old person's problem, arthritis is entering the health scene at a much younger age than in the past. Yet most of us still expect to get poor joints and arthritis as we age. "Aren't we supposed to get arthritis as we age?" There are many people I see with joint pain who when they go to the doctor get told very straight that, "it is your age, and just wear and tear, so either put up with the pain or take anti-inflammatory pain killers". Very rarely do they look into why the pain is there or why have the joints worn so quickly. Even when x-rays show that it is worn, they are told there is nothing that can be done other than medication for the pain, and then at a later date a hip or knee replacement.

I do believe there are some things we can do to reduce the pain using natural methods and supplements, which in turn will also improve the over-all health of the person. There are a few different reasons why someone is likely to have joint pain, so therefore there can be different solutions. Common reasons are; worn cartilage, calcification in the cartilage area, loose cartilage, foreign matter in the joint, damaged ligaments, tendon problems, damaged muscle tissue, joints out of alignment, infections in the joints, excess fluid in the joints, or not enough fluid in the joints.

The most common reason I see for having joint problems is a lack of pressure of the joint fluid; the synovial fluid. The synovial membranes along with the joint ligaments are responsible for holding our synovial fluid under high pressure so as to cushion the contact of the cartilages. Typically when we sprain a joint we are stretching or damaging the ligaments so much that the pressure drops in the fluid. It is a lack of pressure that creates most of the common discomfort experienced by many of us.

When the pressure is low it is very normal to feel a discomfort or pain at times when we are inactive, mainly after sleeping, driving, or sitting for long periods. Once we are up and moving again the pain usually reduces, only to come back again when we are resting. This can sometimes go on for many years and is the prelude to arthritis and worn joints. The first joints to be affected are usually the knees, hips and lower back or any other joint that has had high use such as a carpenter's hammer hand and arm.

When the synovial joint pressure is lower than optimum it is likely that the cartilage will wear very quickly. It is the number one reason our cartilage will wear out, and if the joint alignment is incorrect the cartilage will wear unevenly. The pressure of the fluid in the joints will get low if the ligaments are weaker than required. The ligaments hold the joints together, so if ligaments are weak it is likely the joints will not be in the perfect position, or will be easily moved in and out of alignment. The lack of cushioning between the joints can also lead to the nerves in and around the joints getting pinched when we move in a particular way. This can create intense sudden pain.

Having low pressure in the joint fluid is a very common problem and to my knowledge there is no test available to see just what the pressure of your joint fluid is. The liver is the main controller of this synovial pressure. If we have poor liver function we will always end up with a very acidic body. Check out the chapter on the liver. This acid is very damaging on the ligaments and synovial membrane. They become weaker which means the pressure cannot be held at the correct level.

However this is not the main issue. The main reason for low joint pressure is very poor digestion that results from having a poor liver function. This will always result in the colon functioning very poorly. Near the top of the ascending colon is where we absorb glucosamine sulphate from our food. This glucosamine is very important for complete joint health especially the ligaments and the cartilage repair. If we cannot absorb enough of this glucosamine because of a poor digestive track over a long period of time, the joint pressure will slowly reduce which will result in a very gradual increase in the joint discomfort. This usually takes many months or years so is often just seen as aging.

Because it is a slow and gradual increase in discomfort people easily accept the issue as just aging so do very little to solve the problem, until the pain gets to a point that it is interfering with their lifestyle. The next option for many is pain killer medication and anti-inflammatory, which in most cases helps get rid of the pain but very seldom gets to the real cause of the problem. Natural supplements can work well for some but for many it does little more than hold the progression of the problem, which is great, but once again it is not getting right to the cause.

Joint alignment is a major problem for many, usually a result of accidents, sports injury or common slips in around the home. This can create joint pain that is hard to detect via x-ray or scans. If joints are out of alignment they are likely to wear unevenly creating big problems later in life. Our bone skeleton is the thing that holds us up-right and rigid, but it is the muscles that hold the bones in place.

If joints or bones are not in correct alignment the muscles will usually accommodate by pulling tighter in the effected area, creating discomfort. If the kidney function is poor we will nearly always become de-hydrated which is bad for muscles. The muscles get very tight when de-hydrated which can further increase the discomfort. If muscle tension is not balanced it is easy for the skeleton to get pulled out of position, especially the pelvic area. Massage can give temporary relief but if the muscles stay de-hydrated and or the joints are not well aligned the discomfort will soon return. The muscle will not relax. At this point a good Osteopath or Physiotherapist is worth their weight in gold. A good Osteopath will deal with the skeleton and bone positions as well as muscle tension.

When the fluid pressure is low the body will many times try and fix the problem by putting more fluid into the joint. We see this clearly in our hands and knees. The pressure is low because the ligaments are weak, so if the body keeps putting more fluid into the joint the weak ligaments will continue to stretch. The body is doing the best it can but what are really needed are stronger ligaments, not more fluid.

High levels of quality glucosamine are required to get the synovial pressure back up to the correct level. We will require a higher level of glucosamine for the repair stage compared with maintenance.

It is very important to get the digestion operating well so that we can absorb all the required nutrients for good joint health, both from our food and our supplements. It is very important to understand the digestive system and how it plays such a critical role in good joint health. Too often people do not get the full benefit of joint supplements because the digestion is poor.

Also, we need to have a healthy liver so as to get the correct pH level in our body. In our younger years when the digestion is more efficient we can get enough joint food from our diet to maintain good joint health. As we age we will not be able to get enough for maintenance and even worse, if we injure the joint area, it is near impossible to get enough of the right nutrients for complete repair while still maintaining all the other joints.

So a simple recipe for joint problems is;
- Take a quality glucosamine supplement
- Take a quality omega 3 oil for circulation
- Ensure that the digestion is at the best level possible
- Have ginger tea so as to get the liver functioning well

These are very simple things to do that should have a very positive effect on most joint problems. For spinal discomforts it would be advisable to see a good Osteopath.

EMOTIONAL VS MENTAL

This is a very confusing topic, so therefore a very challenging issue to deal with. What is the difference between emotional and mental and how much of a cross-over is there between them? I will try to answer this in my usual simple, uncomplicated way and hope it makes some kind of sense for you.

There are many differences between emotional and mental, and there are many different forms of each. I am in no way going to get to the bottom of any of these problems in one short chapter, but I do want to share with you some of the everyday situations I see with mental and emotional happenings that could have an effect on the physical body. Negative emotional problems have the capacity to negatively affect the physical body and produce negative physical symptoms, whereas with mental problems it is usually the opposite. An unhealthy body will make mental issues harder to deal with.

In most cases the brain deals with mental issues while emotional issues are very much connected to the liver, but sometimes end up in the brain, just as the mental issues can turn emotional and affect the liver. The most important thing I want to share with you on this topic is the fact that if there is a negative emotional happening in our lives, that stays attached to the body, it will nearly always attach to the liver. This attachment then becomes something like a physical attachment, a leech, and so it can very much affect the physical function of the liver. I touched on this in the chapter on the liver.

If the liver function gets very low and stays poor for a few years, the acidity level in the body will be very poor. This acidity will speed up the rate of degeneration of our cells. Some studies are now showing a very strong link between high acidity levels and cancer. Every cancer patient I have seen has had a very acidic body. From my measuring it is easy to trace most cancer problems back several years or more to a bad emotional happening in that person's life. It may have been a death of a close family member or friend, someone close leaving, a personal grievance fight, a sudden accident or near death experience, or major relationship problems. It can be anything that has a big emotional component.

At the time of the incident it will nearly always affect the liver, but for some of us that effect will subdue over the next few weeks and have no long-term effects. For others it will stay attached to the liver like a leech and after a few months start to have a negative effect on the physical function of the liver.

Poor liver function effects the acid levels throughout our body and so on it goes. This is a very common and very real issue for many people in any society. Emotional problems cause cancer. There is a lot of evidence that chemicals and cancers are linked. The liver is the detox centre of our body, so if the liver is low because of emotional problems it will be easier for chemicals to get into our cells and do their damage. The poor liver function is also very damaging on the digestive system which will result in nutrient deficiencies, which are also very closely connected with cancer and many other degenerative diseases.

So you can see how having an emotional attachment in your body can very directly create serious degenerative disease. And it is all very easy to avoid. There are many things that are good for the liver but the best simple thing I know is ginger tea. You have to use fresh root ginger. Just cut a small slice of ginger off the root and place it in a cup, then poor on the boiling water. Do not microwave the tea. You can drink it hot or cold, but it has to be made hot to be effective. In the first 2-3 days it is worth while having up to three cups a day. After that, one cup daily is fine.

Another option is to make up a strong cup of ginger tea and when it has cooled down pour it into your drink bottle, top it up with cold water and then consume it throughout the day. This tea is usually very good at controlling emotional issues as we live through them and also very good at detaching any emotional problems that have been holding onto your liver for a long period. Please try this ginger tea, it can help in numerous ways and the taste is very refreshing.

Mental problems are quite different in that they are more to do with everyday worries like being over worked or financial problems or worrying about other people's problems, especially family members. This is a very large problem covering many different issues, but what I want to high-light is the fact that the brain is the part of the body that deals with mental problems.

Also, there is a big difference between having a mental disease and being mentally stressed. There is also a big difference between being depressed and having depression. Mental disease is primarily where there is a chemical imbalance in the brain that has a negative effect on brain function. It controls you. Sometimes genetics will also play a roll here. This is a field I don't intend to deal with at this time. What I want to cover briefly is the over all health of your brain cell.

The brain has two main functions; one being it deals with

intellectual, learning, memory and information type things. The second function of the brain is that it is the computer that keeps your body functioning. It has the ability to look after each and every cell in your body. It does not have to be trained to do this; it just knows everything that is required to make every organ and system in your body work in perfect harmony so long as all things are in place at the cellular level. It is beyond comprehension just how brilliant your brain is at keeping your body functioning, and the most amazing thing of all is that it did not require any programming at any stage in your life. Right from the start of your life, your brain just knew what to do. It is a very complicated electrical object that does not need to be told what to do. It just does it.

There is one very important thing that your brain does need though, and that is food. By food I mean several different things that are needed to feed the brain cells so that they can do their function, mainly oxygen, water and nutrients. If your brain cell is not getting enough of these foods it will not be able to work at full capacity. A brain cell that is lacking in oxygen, fluid, and nutrients will not be able to think or learn properly. It will struggle with information recall, long term memory but especially short term memory. Our ability to learn information will be below our natural capabilities. Many learning disabilities are closely associated with a low level of nutrients in the brain cell.

What I am covering here is just an extension of the food, digestion, liver and kidney issues, but I am hoping you will see how it has a very direct impact on the brain function. How can a brain cell function well if it is not fed all the nutrients it requires?

Compare it to your leg muscle. If that muscle has used up most of its oxygen and nutrients it will not work well and so needs a rest. In severe cases the muscle will start cramping. A brain cell is no different. If it is not fed properly how can it function properly? How can it be efficient at information storage and how can it function the rest of the body properly?

If a cell is under nourished there is a greater chance that chemicals and toxins will enter that cell. Many mental health problems, particularly Alzheimer's, have been shown to have connections with heavy metals, toxins and chemicals. Just because a body is exposed to chemicals does not mean it will be negatively affected by them. What matters is whether the chemicals get into our cells. If a cell is fully fed it is very hard for toxins and chemicals to get into it and do any damage. I am not talking here about some short term issue that just happened last week. No, it is a life long issue. The brain cells need to be fully feed with quality nutrients, oxygen and water they require for life long full function.

I have seen many children with learning difficulties, ADD or ADHD who are very low in nutrients in the brain cell area. It was mentioned earlier about the liver and acidic problems. When the acid level gets bad it has a very negative impact on how efficient our brain cells will work. This acidity is usually connected with emotional problems, so now you should be able to see how emotional problems can affect the brain function because of this acid problem, and then up come the mental problems.

Emotional problems can sometimes be the very reason we have mental problems. Also check back in the kidney chapter to see how poor kidney function can have a very negative affect on brain function. A very common symptom for bad kidneys is short term memory problems and de-hydrated brain cells.

Blood is our life line. It is blood that transports things around the body for us, taking the good things to the cells and then taking the rubbish out. If blood quality is poor or the ability of the blood to flow through our blood vessels is restricted, it will have a negative affect on the cell function. I covered this in the heart chapter.

Ginkgo is frequently used when there are brain function problems. The main function of ginkgo is to stimulate brain blood vessels to expand so more blood can flow through to nourish the brain cells. Ginkgo can be helpful if circulation is an issue. Also, high doses of omega 3 fish oils and flaxseed oils are recommended. These oils can clean out the blood vessels so as to let more blood through. The omega 3 is good to help repair and stimulate nerves in the brain.

One thing that is hard to measure is the electrical connections between brain cells. It has been estimated that there are about 10,000 electrical connections coming from each brain cell that connect with other brain cells. I don't know how they counted them but regardless of the exact number, it is beyond understanding. Having poor electrical connections between brain cells is a common reason why a brain is functioning poorly. This poor communication between brain cells will slow down the brain. It is however very easily improved with an herbal tincture made from gotu kola. For most people it will require about 10 days of taking gotu kola to get your brain cell communication working faster. If the brain is working faster it can help improve many different body functions.

Tied up with all of this is the possibility of having a long term viral infection in the brain area. Once again check out the chapter on viruses. In many cases I deal with, there is usually more than one reason for poor brain function. There is nearly always a combination of several of the reasons that have been mentioned in this chapter. I see it this way. The brain cell will not be able to function fully because it is either too polluted, undernourished due to either poor blood or poor circulation, has an infection, is very acidic, or is not sleeping on a good spot. There are many other reasons why the brain function may be poor but those just mentioned will cover most cases.

Sleep can play a big part with brain function. Read closely the sleep chapter to understand the enormous amount of work your brain is trying to do at sleep time. The brain cell needs a perfect exterior environment as well as a perfect environment in the cell for it to do the sleep process correctly. Because the brain is somewhat similar to muscles we need to treat it similar by giving it some healthy stimulation on a regular basis. Use it or lose it.

Now, a growing issue with the 'use it or lose it' is the fact that some people are giving the brain too much information and creating an over-load. This is very common when a person is very unwell. They will not know what is wrong and their doctor is unable to come up with a clear diagnosis, so they get on the internet and get a wealth of information about their symptoms.

This provides them with huge amounts of information that is very interesting and sounds very correct in relation to their symptoms. Many times confusion enters their thoughts at this time because of this information over-load. This is because a lot of the information they have found will read correct and seem appropriate to their condition, but may not be relevant. The brain cannot always work out the difference between wrong and right.

If there is too much information it can find it very hard to differentiate between what is relevant or not. All of the information may be correct but most of it may not be relevant to their health issue. The brain is the computer that functions the body. If you have too much information in the computer or have information that the computer does not know whether it is relevant or not, it could cause the computer to work wrong.

Over programming of the brain will confuse the brain as to how it is supposed to be functioning. Figuring out what is relevant is the most important task, and the brain will find this hard if there is too much information that is technically correct and that sounds appropriate to the health problem. Sometimes it is a very fine line between what is appropriate or not and it is hard to know where this line is.

For many people this information over-load creates a situation where they are trying to make life happen rather than just letting it happen. In other words, we need to listen to our intuitive instincts as versus using information to make the body work a particular way. Get on with life and try to trust that thing inside us that can guide us in the right direction. Get in tune with it and let it get involved in your life, but don't always try and analyse it so as to understand it. Just trust it. Remember, the simplest solutions are many times the best solutions.

So whether we just have some minor short term memory problems, difficulty with decision making, mental worry over family issues and money or serious mental health problems, we can all benefit from feeding our brain cells with the optimum level of quality nutrients. I hope you can now see there is a difference between mental and emotional issues, yet at the same time how some of them are the same and how emotional issues can have a very controlling influence over mental function because of the livers effect on acidity.

But the biggest thing to learn from all of this is that the brain is still just one part of the whole body and is very much affected by how other systems are working and lifestyle choices. Too often medical people don't see the brain as a physical object, just like a muscle, and therefore treat it as if it is something other than physical. A lot of people with mental health problems only ever get offered treatments that revolve around chemical prescriptions and talking/counselling.

If we could see it more as a solid object and try and find solutions that suit it as a solid matter, especially nutrients, then I know we would experience some good lasting solutions. In most cases of people with brain type problems it is very likely that the health professional will only be looking at the brain itself and very seldom looks at other organs or systems. Many times the liver and or kidneys are the only reason for brain function problems.

We have all heard the statement "Healthy mind, healthy body". Well the opposite of that is also true. "Healthy body, healthy mind".

CHAPTER THIRTEEN
BASIC GUIDELINES

This is a summary of all the solutions I have mentioned earlier, and there will be a few extras. When we look at health problems and try to find solutions in the herbal or natural foods area all the selections are somewhat overwhelming. Which ones work, which ones don't, which one will suit me best and just how are you supposed to use that particular herb? Oh, so many questions and such confusion. There has been a library of books written on the subject, some short, precise and uncomplicated, while others have more than one thousand pages of extremely interesting information, most of which it true, but how can one know what is relevant or not.

When we have too many choices on any particular topic, people will pick one of two very common options. First option is they will do nothing because there is too much confusion or the second option is they will do the same thing they have always done. The best option is that they will try something different but only if someone can educate them as to which is the best option to take.

In most situations in life we now have too many choices which are only creating confusion. It is well proven that confused people usually do nothing. In most situations we need simple solutions that people can understand and achieve without having to change their lifestyle too drastically. From my experience in the health work I do, in most cases you can be sure that there are simple solutions that will work very well, and the client will experience a very clear and permanent improvement in symptoms.

There are two basic types of solutions. The first is something that will give an immediate relief of symptoms. The second will be dealing more with long term problems and permanent long term improvements. Short term solutions usually revolve around some type of pain killer, anti inflammatory, antibiotic medicine, either chemical based or natural plant based.

Suggested long term solutions will many times require a person to make major lifestyle changes, especially with dietary and exercise programmes. While this is very good it will require a person to make sacrifices that are hard, and they will have to force themselves to stick to the suggested programme. With perseverance this will usually work but it takes a lot of time and hard effort that is not always enjoyable or fun.

However, I have seen too many such cases where the person does not get the desired improvements; especially in the weight loss area. This will be because they have not got to the core reason for the health problem, which in many cases will be the digestion, liver or kidneys. What I have found in most cases is there will be a small thing we need to do so as to make the body feel better. This trigger will give the body its own self belief that it can heal. The body will then want to get better because it has had a quick taste of improvement and actually now knows it can function better, as versus many of the long term suggested solutions, which will force the body to change. When the body gets a small taste of this quick improvement it will take you to better things such as better dietary choices and lifestyle options.

Let me give just a few simple things that we can all do with safety that should help to ensure the main basic functions of the body are working well. The three most common areas of concern are the digestion, kidneys, and liver.

For all of us we need to get our digestion working better. We all could benefit from a few weeks of root ginger tea for the liver function and add to that some fresh parsley for the kidneys. Everyone should be taking a quality omega 3 oil, so as to help circulation. If you feel your sleep is not as refreshing as it should be then try sleeping somewhere else.

Your food selection should be mainly about plants. Source foods that are fresh alive plants and then make sure you don't over-cook or kill this food. Anything animal should represent only a small portion of your total food. The foods you eat should taste good for you. Just because someone else might like asparagus doesn't mean you have to like it. There are many, many different foods to select from. Find fresh, alive food that tastes good for you and make sure you eat enough of it. The most critical thing of all with food is not how good the quality of the food is, but whether that food actually gets to the cells of your body to nourish them. So get your digestion operating at a healthy level. Then savor the moment, food should be fun.

Be proactive about physical exercise. It does not have to be all about a hard work out at the gym. What is needed is regular exercise that you enjoy and even have fun doing. It is the same as with food. If you know a particular form of exercise is very good for you but you don't like doing that type of exercise, then don't do it. But make sure you do find an exercise routine that you do enjoy. If you can have genuine fun while you exercise it will nearly double the value of that exercise.

There are plenty of options to choose from. There is no excuse for not getting some form of physical movement on a regular basis. Even when you are sitting in your chair you can do some arm movement. I have an 87 year old gentleman friend, who on awaking each morning will kick the blankets of his bed, lie there and do 30 leg lifts before getting out of his bed. If you do have a reason for not exercising regularly then can I politely suggest you are just lazy? If you look after your body, it will thank you in so many ways.

You may be one of the many millions of people around the world suffering from one of our common degenerative diseases of cancer, cardiovascular disease, MS, chronic fatigue, diabetes, arthritis, osteoporosis, Alzheimer's or obesity. Or you may fall into the category of people who are just tired and run-down, always low on energy and have lost the zest for life. Or you may feel great and have no health problems that you can see or feel. Either way I encourage you to take seriously the information I have shared with you.

Many years ago I started to learn how to listen to the human body and over these ensuing years I have tried to develop that listening skill. There have been thousands of bodies that I have listened to. They have told me most of what I have written in this book. The body does know how to talk to us about health issues. We have to learn how to listen and understand the body's language. It will not lie to us about our health. I have many times seen enormous improvements in a person's health when all they did was try some very simple solution for some very complex problems.

Be not concerned about who the messenger is or how they received the information. Just look at the information and see if it is logical and relevant. Do not presume that just because your health feels good that it is. Degenerative diseases can develop over many years and take hold in our body long before we feel any clear symptoms. We all need to be more pro-active about our health rather than reactive. Don't wait until something goes wrong before you act. Too many of us have very clear symptoms to tell us that our body is not functioning well and yet choose to ignore it. We presume it is supposed to feel this way because of our age or stage of life. Don't be fooled. If the body tells you it is not feeling well it will nearly always be because of an internal function problem rather than something outside of the body that we might call 'life'.

Please go back to the start of this book and read the quote from James M. Carroll in the introduction.

We have been blessed with a fantastic vehicle to live in while we are on this Earth. It is a very special sacred vessel. Enjoy it and have fun with it but most of all give it respect and love. It is the only one you have. If it is looked after correctly it will give you many years of quality use, free of degeneration and pain and allow the spirit living within it to completely flourish to its full potential.

CHAPTER FOURTEEN
SUPPLEMENTATION

Should we take supplements, and if we do, which ones should we take? How do we know the good supplements from the bad ones?

The answer for the first question is no. We shouldn't take supplements, because if we eat properly we should be able to get all the nutrients we require for optimum long term health. Nature can provide us with all we need if we grow the right food and eat the correct amount of these quality plants.

However, for most of us it is nearly impossible to receive all the required nutrients from our food. The quality of the foods we purchase is way below what is needed for today's health issues. Most of the foods we eat are seriously depleted of the vital minerals, vitamins and antioxidants that are needed, especially the processed foods.

Therefore, the correct answer to the first question is yes, most of us do need to take some form of supplementation so as to make up for the shortfall in the food we are eating. Many studies have clearly shown the benefits of taking good supplements. When most of us are spending many years of our life suffering from a degenerative disease we need to ask the question why. Studies have also shown that a lack of some core nutrients at the cellular level is a major contributing factor for many of these common degenerative diseases we face.

In many cases quality supplements can help to improve health conditions. What is more important for me though, is taking a quality supplement so as to avoid getting unwell. It is easier to avoid getting some degenerative diseases than what it is to fix them once you have the problem.

Choosing a quality supplement is not easy. How can the average consumer determine what is a quality supplement or not? There is too much choice in the market place. This will create confusion. Confused customers will either do the same old thing over and over or they will do nothing. Supplement consumers need to get informed, unbiased information. This is not easy to get.

A quality supplement will be manufactured at a pharmaceutical standard and carry a 100% guarantee of quality, purity and potency. Our first option should be to take a multi vitamin and mineral supplement. Give the body everything it needs and let it decide what is needed. How can we really know whether we need more calcium and vitamin B12 as versus magnesium and iron? We don't know. So give your cells everything and let them decide. A very common criticism of supplements is that 'we are just peeing all that money and nutrients down the toilet'. I would rather pee a dollar down the toilet each day than be 10 cents short of what is needed. This accumulated shortfall over many years will starve your cells of vital nutrients required for optimum health. Avoiding a problem is much cheaper than trying to fix it later. We need to be pro-active not re-active.

In an ideal world we would not need supplements, but the reality of today is that supplementation is essential for long-term optimum health. The problem is not just about the lack of goodness in our foods, but also the high level of oxidative stress we are placing on our bodies due to our poor life-style choices and work place environments. Quality supplements can give a high level of anti-oxidant protection against many degenerative problems.

So be pro-active and invest in quality supplements that can help your body in many ways both now and in the future. Your body will thank you for it.

If you want to keep your body alive put alive plants into it.

Some Simple Solutions
Fresh root ginger tea – *Liver problems*
> Emotional issues
> Indigestion
> Reflux and wind
> Eczema
> Safe to have on a regular basis.

Parsley tea – *Kidney problems*
> Dark under eyes
> Always tired
> Skin pimples and boils
> Always cold with poor circulation
> Safe to have on a regular basis.

Chives tea – *Bacterial infections in the digestion, kidneys, bladder, or blood.*
> Have maximum of five cups at any time.

Sage tea – *Metabolism and hormonal issues*
> Have maximum of five cups at any time.

Rosemary tea – *Good for hydration*
   Tight muscles
   Constipation
   Have no more than six cups at any time.

Thyme tea – *Good for fungal infections*
   As a tea to drink and a skin wash

Omega3 oil – *either fish oil or flaxseed*
   Cleans out fatty plaque deposits in blood vessels
   Essential for heart disease patients

Ginger and sage tea combined *will kill most common virus.*
   Do not exceed 6 cups at any given time.

Gotukola is very good for slow brain function.

ABOUT THE AUTHOR

Kevin was born into a farming family in rural New Zealand. From the earliest age he had a passion for agricultural activity and understanding of how nature really works. In his last year of education he achieved the highest levels in biology that had been seen for many years. His understanding of biological matters was evident at a very young age. Not one to openly question the system, Kevin worked quietly but surely to get connected with nature so as to understand how the biology of life functions. He was and still is rather frustrated at how science has become too complicated and thus confuse things. For Kevin Science has been wearing two hats. One hat represents the situation where Science has come up with discoveries that have revolutionized our understanding of health, and this is just fantastic. The advancements in human health have been huge. The other hat is a very negative hat to wear because it says that if Science can't understand or explain something, it is not true. If Science does not approve it then it is scorned.

Kevin is now a natural health consultant living and working from his home in New Plymouth, New Zealand. With his wife of 30 years, Glenis, he has a grown family of 4 children. They 'walk the talk', living in an environmentally friendly home on 16 acres of organically farmed land producing most of their food requirements. 25 years ago Kevin started his health quest by studying Bau Biology and Ecology. This is a study of how the built environment can affect our health (biology) and how it might affect the ecology of the planet. Since then he has used the skill of radiesthesia to measure the human body so as to see why it is not functioning fully. The significant improvement in his patients health situation has been the driving force which has allowed his work to spread to all corners of this planet. He never planned or decided to be a health consultant at any stage. It just evolved as a result of people having an improvement in their own personal health.

Kevin is a marathon runner, enjoys long distance cycling, home gardening, is a church man and family man. Within all of this he has a passion for helping people to optimize their health with simple solutions and lifestyle options.

Contact details;
Kevin McDonald
Heartlands
RD 3
New Plymouth
New Zealand
E-mail: heartlands@clear.net.nz

CPSIA information can be obtained at www.ICGtesting.com
231448LV00005B/14/P

9 780473 150457